PROSTHETICS & ORTHOTICS

Donald G. Shurr, CO, PT
Director of External Relations
American Prosthetics, Inc.
Iowa City, Iowa

Thomas M. Cook, PT, PhD
Assistant Professor
Physical Therapy Graduate Program
University of Iowa
Iowa City, Iowa

APPLETON & LANGE
Norwalk, Connecticut

Notice: Our knowledge in clinical sciences is constantly changing.
As new information becomes available, changes in treatment and in the use of drugs
become necessary. The authors and the publisher of this volume have taken
care to make certain that the doses of drugs and schedules of treatment are
correct and compatible with the standards generally accepted at the time of
publication. The reader is advised to consult carefully the instruction
and information material included in the package insert of each drug or
therapeutic agent before administration. This advice is especially
important when using new or infrequently used drugs.

Copyright © 1990 by Appleton & Lange
A Publishing Division of Prentice Hall

93 94 / 10 9 8 7 6 5 4
Prentice Hall International (UK) Limited, *London*
Prentice Hall of Australia Pty. Limited, *Sydney*
Prentice Hall Canada, Inc., *Toronto*
Prentice Hall Hispanoamericana, S.A., *Mexico*
Prentice Hall of India Private Limited, *New Delhi*
Prentice Hall of Japan, Inc., *Tokyo*
Simon & Schuster Asia Pte. Ltd., *Singapore*
Editora Prentice Hall do Brasil Ltda., *Rio de Janeiro*
Prentice Hall, *Englewood Cliffs, New Jersey*

Library of Congress Cataloging-in-Publication Data

Shurr, Donald G.
    Prosthetics and orthotics / by Donald G. Shurr & Thomas M. Cook.
        p. cm.
    ISBN 0-8385-7977-9
    1. Prosthesis.   2. Orthopedic apparatus.   I. Cook, Thomas M.
(Thomas Michael), 1944–   . II. Title.
    [DNLM: 1. Orthotic Devices.   2. Prosthesis.   WE 172 S562p]
RD130.S53   1990
617'.9—dc20
DNLM/DLC
for Library of Congress   89-17650
                                                                          CIP

Acquisitions Editor: Stephany Scott
Production Editor: Louise Whelan
Designer: Janice Barsevich

PRINTED IN THE UNITED STATES OF AMERICA

This book is dedicated to Marilyn, Carrie, Molly, Joan, Jenny, and Jonathan.

It is also dedicated to the unfinished work ahead, begun with one of our mentors, Mr. Harold E. Miller, CPO, whose untimely death did not allow us to learn from him all that he desired to teach, or we to learn.

Contents

Foreword

Too frequently, an amputation is assumed to be the final event in the care of a patient instead of the beginning of a critical phase in functional restoration and improvement of quality of life by the use of modern prosthetic and rehabilitative methods.

Too frequently, adults and children with neuromusculoskeletal disorders have been relegated to a life of disability instead of receiving attempts to overcome impairment by contemporary orthotic and restorative techniques.

This deplorable state of affairs results from two major problems in the education of health professionals: the lack of emphasis on the subject in curricular design and the heretofore absence of a thoughtfully prepared text designed to provide a coordinated overview for the serious student who needs an understandable distillate of an evolving, fragmented, and complex discipline.

The authors of this text deserve congratulations for undertaking the formidable task of helping correct these aberrations. I am honored to have worked with them and I have learned much from them over these past several years. I can attest to their comprehensive knowledge of the subject, their ability to teach, and their tireless dedication to the care of patients.

This inclusive volume with chapters on materials, mechanics, upper and lower limb prosthetics and orthotics, and spinal orthotics presents an overview and a method of approach that reflects, in a superb manner, both the art and science of the subject. It will be of great benefit not only to the beginning student but also to those who want to extend their working knowledge of the fascinating, dynamic, and increasingly important topic of prosthetics and orthotics.

I, and many of my colleagues, express deep appreciation to the authors for their time and effort in providing yet another service to patients through those whose education will be greatly enhanced by this text.

Reginald R. Cooper, MD
Chairman, Department of Orthopaedics
University of Iowa
Iowa City, Iowa

Preface

This volume has been developed while teaching prosthetics and orthotics to entry level physical therapy students over a period of seven years. During that time our students and others have asked us repeatedly to refer them to a single resource around which they could focus their learning. This book is our response to their prodding.

Although developed primarily for physical therapy students, this book should be useful for anyone without experience or background in prosthetics and orthotics. It should be appropriate for other health care professionals such as nurses, physicians, occupational therapists, vocational counselors, and so forth. The text assumes only a basic understanding of anatomy, kinesiology, and, to some extent, pathology.

The primary objective of this volume is to provide a sound overview of the art and science of prosthetics and orthotics as currently practiced in America. We fully recognize that there are distinct regional differences and preferences in P&O practice throughout this country and others. The reader should know that he or she may never encounter some of the devices described in this text and is very likely to encounter devices which vary significantly, or even drastically, from those presented herein. This book is not intended as an encyclopedic treatise of every possible P&O device. Such a work, if possible, would be overwhelming in size and outdated before it appeared in print. Rather, our intention is to address the fundamental concepts underlying the selection and application of common prosthetic and orthotic devices. Our hope is that the interested reader will use this information as a foundation for improving the quality of patient care in whatever setting he or she encounters.

A final comment must be made about the concept of combining both prosthetics and orthotics in one volume. Although traditionally considered as somewhat distinct topics, we have found an integrated approach to teaching these subjects to be very logical and effective. Recent developments in materials and fabrication methods and common functional goals for applying these external devices appear to blur some of the long-standing distinctions between these two disciplines. Perhaps some later edition of this or a similar book might well be entitled "Prosthotics"!

Donald G. Shurr
Thomas M. Cook

Acknowledgments

The preparation of this work was made possible through the unselfish efforts of many people. Thanks are extended to all the physical therapy students over the years who have provided the inspiration and feedback for this work during its various stages of development. We also thank Dr. Maurice Schnell, Dr. R. R. Cooper, Ben Wilson, Melvin Stills, CO, and Charles Pritham, CPO, for the interest they engendered in this field and for the hours they spent sharing their knowledge with us. We are also indebted to our colleagues at American Prosthetics, Inc., and at the University of Iowa for their tolerance and support in this endeavor. We especially appreciate the untiring efforts, patience, and attention to detail provided by Judy Biderman and Carol Lipsius during the seemingly endless revisions of the manuscript. Finally, we recognize the invaluable contributions of the patients, who have taught us far more than we have taught them.

CHAPTER 1

Introduction to Prosthetics and Orthotics

This chapter will present a brief historical perspective on the development of the fields of orthotics and prosthetics followed by a description of orthotic and prosthetic services as currently provided in the United States. Overviews of prosthetics and orthotics include discussions of those factors common to all amputees and users of orthotic devices. The chapter includes a description of the prosthetics/orthotics clinic team.

HISTORICAL PERSPECTIVE

Brief History of Prosthetics

Historically amputation was often the only medical alternative in the definitive treatment of complex fractures or infections of the extremities. Although even Neolithic man was thought to have the necessary knowledge and tools to accomplish amputations, many patients most likely did not survive the procedure. By the sixth century BC, the physician Susruta wrote detailed works about proper surgical procedure that became standard technique. The more precise the procedure and the faster the amputations were done, the higher the survival rates.

Early prosthetists were blacksmiths, armor makers, other skilled artisans, and the patients themselves. Early limbs manufactured in Europe and later in America used metal, wood, and leather. Articulated knee and ankle joints eventually replaced stiff joints, and gradually metal was replaced by wood. These changes made the devices more functional and lighter in weight.

In 1860 A.A. Marks substituted a hard rubber foot for a wooden one. Soon after, J.E. Hanger, an amputee in the Confederate army, placed rubber bumpers in solid feet and thus produced the first articulated prosthetic feet. Hanger also popularized skin suction as a method of suspending an above-knee prosthesis. Prosthetics grew tremendously during the Civil War, as over 30,000 amputations were performed on the Union side alone. Wooden socket limbs from Marks of New York sold at that time for $75 to $150 each and were available by mail order.

War continued to provide the major impetus for research and development in prosthetics. Details and materials have changed considerably since 1900, but little change has occurred in the basic designs of limb prosthetics. Following World War II, the Veteran's Administration (VA) financially supported the development of the patellar-tendon bearing and quadrilateral sockets for below-knee and above-knee amputees, respectively. These designs and techniques were taught to all prosthetists so that both veteran and civilian amputees would benefit. Following Vietnam, renewed funding by the VA led to further refinements in prostheses, including the provision of myoelectrically controlled upper-extremity prostheses and endoskeletal, modular prostheses.

Brief History of Orthotics

The development of the art and science of splinting and bracemaking, now referred to as the field of orthotics, very much paralleled developments in the field of prosthetics. Pictorial examples of splints and various assistive devices can be found among early civilizations, including ancient Egyptians and Greeks. The same materials, metal, leather, and wood, found in early prosthetic devices were also used in orthotic devices; and the same artisans, namely, blacksmiths, armor makers, and patients, were the first orthotists.

By the 18th and 19th centuries the manufacture of thin steel had reached such a refined state that splints and braces were sometimes mass produced and described in catalogues often published by enterprising "appliance makers." Pioneers in this early period were Ambroise Pare (1509–1590); Hugh Owen Thomas (1834–1901); and Sir Robert Jones, a nephew of Hugh Owen Thomas, who is considered to be the "father of orthopaedic surgery." All were accomplished and innovative bracemakers as well as "bonesetters." Eventually surgery replaced manipulation and bracing as the cornerstone of the practice of orthopaedics. Bracemakers then became professionals distinct from physicians.

The term *orthotics* has recently replaced the use of the word *bracing* to describe the control of body segments by external devices. *Orthotics* is meant to include dynamic control of body segments compared to the more limited, static connotations of the word "brace." The term was first used in the early 1950s and was originally adopted in 1960 by orthotists and prosthetists in America when they formed the American Orthotic and Prosthetic Association from the original Artificial Limb Manufacturers' Association.

Just as the wars of this century have caused a renewed interest in the development of prosthetics, the polio epidemics of the 1950s spurred increased interest in the field of orthotics. Beginning around 1970, many innovations in orthotic designs were made possible by the adaptation of industrial techniques for vacuum-forming sheet plastics. Because of the continuing introduction of new materials and methods, present-day orthotics practice is a growing, rapidly changing discipline.

PROSTHETIC AND ORTHOTIC SERVICES

Need for Services

The National Health Interview Survey[1] published in 1969 indicated that those using prosthetic legs numbered 0.6 per thousand. By 1977[2] the figures had jumped to one per thousand using an artificial leg. Total people reported to be using either artificial legs or arms in 1977 were 275,000.

For the same population survey, 6,250,000 people in America used orthoses, wheelchairs, canes, or special shoes in 1969.[3] By 1977[2] the number had grown to 6,500,000, or about 3% of the American population. Specifically, people using leg orthoses increased from 233,000 in 1969 to 400,000 in 1977. This represents roughly 1.2 people per thousand population in 1969 and 1.9 people per thousand in 1977, nearly twice the number using prostheses.

Professional Organization and Certification

Certification of both professionals and facilities is administered by the American Board for Certification (ABC) in Orthotics and Prosthetics, Inc. This board was established in 1948 through a combined effort of the orthotics and prosthetics industry and the American Academy of Orthopaedic Surgeons. The ABC promotes high professional standards and high-quality facilities and develops and administers examinations in prosthetics and orthotics. Additionally, the organization serves as an appeals committee for alleged violations of established standards of practice, ethics, or law.

Educational Programs

There are currently 10 practitioner-level programs located in the United States.[4] In addition, there are three technician, or assistant-level, programs. Using the enrollment figures published in *Orthotics and Prosthetics*, 184 students will graduate per year from these 10 schools. There are five approved residencies and one master's degree program. It should be noted that other students come from the Army orthotic school, whose model differs from most others in that no formal education is required prior to admission. According to the current standards of ABC, graduates of this program do not qualify to sit for the orthotics board examination and therefore will not increase the credentialed work force in the field for the future.

Currently there is only one subprofessional in orthotics and prosthetics, the technician.[5] Technician education programs are certified by ABC, and technicians are registered as opposed to being certified.

Number and Distribution of Prosthetists and Orthotists

Since 1949 there have been more than 880 prosthetist/orthotists (CPO), 1,392 orthotists (CO), and 1,232 prosthetists (CP) certified by the ABC in Prosthetics and Orthotics, Inc. On July 1, 1982 there were 817 COs, 739 CPs, and 580 CPOs in good standing.[6] This total of 2,136 represented the current certified work force in orthotics and prosthetics (Fig. 1–1). Assuming the present total of 2,136 professionals, together with an

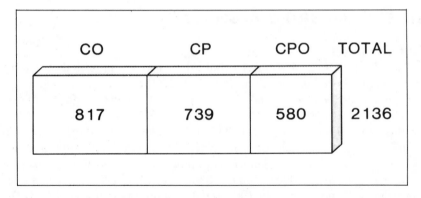

Figure 1–1. Numbers of certified orthotists and prosthetists in the United States in 1982 (CO = certified orthotist; CP = certified prosthetist; CPO = certified prosthetist/orthotist). (From Shurr DG. The delivery of orthotic and prosthetic services in the US—a physical therapist's view. *Orthot Prosthet* 1984; **38**:57, with permission.)

addition of 9% to 10% per year for eight years, and 1% to 2% annual retirement rate, by 1990 there will be approximately 4,000 orthotic/prosthetic practitioners in America. This is in contrast to 560,000 physicians, 2 million nurses, and 40,000 physical therapists (Table 1–1).

At this time in the United States, orthotists and prosthetists practice in five major settings. The first and most common of these settings is the private office. Beginning in the late 1880s,[7] orthotists began moving out of physicians' offices and hospitals in an effort to be independent providers of services and devices and to avail such services to many physicians and patients.

The second commonest practice setting for the delivery of prosthetic and orthotic services is the institutionally based service/consultation. Many large institutions such as hospitals, particularly children's hospitals, rehabilitation centers, and rehabilitation and research institutes provide orthotic/prosthetic services from an internal staff.

The third type of practice in which a prosthetist/orthotist might be involved is that of a supplier and fabrication manager. The use of a central production laboratory, which is physically different from the site of measuring and fitting, has grown rapidly in recent years and will probably continue to increase in America. The economic and professional advantages and disadvantages of this type of arrangement will be discussed more fully in Chapter 2.

TABLE 1–1. PROJECTIONS OF HEALTH CARE PROFESSIONALS IN 1990

Registered nurse (RN)	2,000,000
Physician	560,000
Physician (orthopaedic surgeon)	17,500
CP/CO/CPO	4,000
Physical therapist	40,000

From Shurr DG. The delivery of orthotic and prosthetic services in the US—a physical therapist's view. Orthot Prosthet *1984;* **38***:57, with permission.*

In the 10 programs available for orthotic or prosthetic entry-level preparation, there are full-time professional faculty responsible for this education. According to a 1976 report,[5] there were 17 full-time certified prosthetists, 24 full-time certified orthotists, and 13 full-time certified prosthetists/orthotists in this area of practice.

Finally, few, if any, individuals work in America today doing only basic research in orthotics/prosthetics. This does not, however, include those practitioners who are working on the cutting edge of materials, design, or rehabilitation engineering as part of their daily clinical practice.

The Prosthetics/Orthotics Clinic Team

Due to the complexity of many prosthetic/orthotic cases, referral is often made to a clinic team. Included on this team are likely to be the physician, prosthetist/orthotist, nurse, physical therapist, social worker, vocational counselor, and, most importantly, *the patient*. It is impossible for this clinic team to function meaningfully without the contributions of the patient.

Clinic teams provide evaluation, prescription, delivery, and follow-up prosthetic/orthotic services. Follow-up is important, since the possibility of changes in either the device or the patient necessitate regular re-evaluation by the experienced team. This is extremely important when caring for children, as growth and configuration may change rapidly, requiring concomitant changes in the prosthesis or orthosis. All devices demand some maintenance or replacement and for that reason should be evaluated regularly for proper function.

AN OVERVIEW OF LIMB PROSTHETICS

The term amputation refers to the process whereby a part is severed from the body. The term prosthesis refers to an artificial device used to replace a missing part of the body. The portion of the limb that remains intact following the amputation is referred to as the residual limb, or stump, and the portion of the prosthesis that is fitted over the residual limb is called the prosthetic socket. With proper care the amputee (the individual who has undergone an amputation) can return to a useful life, and amputees can be found in nearly every occupation. When the proper surgical techniques have been employed and when sound training methods and devices are used in providing the prosthesis, the amputee can be expected to participate in many of his or her previous activities.

The Amputee Population

Figures 1–2 and 1–3 summarize statistics on the relative incidence of amputation as reported by Kay and Newman in 1975.[8] Figure 1–2 shows the relative distribution of amputees by site of amputation, and it is clear that the large majority of amputations occur in the lower extremities. As a general rule, it is estimated that there are about 11 lower limb amputees for every upper limb amputee.[8] Figure 1–3 shows the distribution

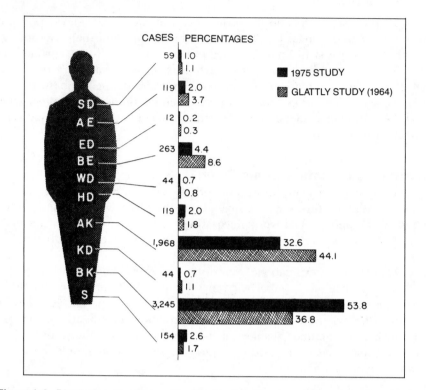

Figure 1–2. Distribution of amputees by site of amputation, comparing studies done in 1975 with 1964 (SD = shoulder disarticulation; AE = above elbow; ED = elbow disarticulation; BE = below elbow; WD = wrist disarticulation; HD = hip disarticulation; AK = above knee; KD = knee disarticulation; BK = below knee; S = Syme's). (From Kay HW, Newman JD. Relative incidence of new amputations. *Orthot Prosthet* 1975; **29**:8, with permission.)

of amputees by sex and cause of amputation. It can be seen that the leading cause of amputation is vascular disease, with an approximate equal incidence between males and females. It is also clear that most vascular amputations occur to people aged 61 to 70 years, with approximately equal occurrence in ages 51 to 60 years and 71 to 80 years.

Level of Amputation

Amputation may occur through joints or through bone. In general, the site of amputation is described by the joint or nearest joint through which the amputation has been made. Common descriptors of sites of amputation are shown in Figure 1–2. An amputation of the lower limb makes standing and walking difficult, while an amputation of the upper limb poses a different set of problems related to activities of daily living (ADL).

Causes of Amputation

Causes of amputation may be grouped into four major categories: trauma, disease, tumor, and congenital. Amputation may be the result of trauma or the result of a life-saving surgical procedure intended to arrest a disease. Additionally, a small percentage of individuals are born without a limb or limbs or with defective limbs that require surgical conversion to a more appropriate level.

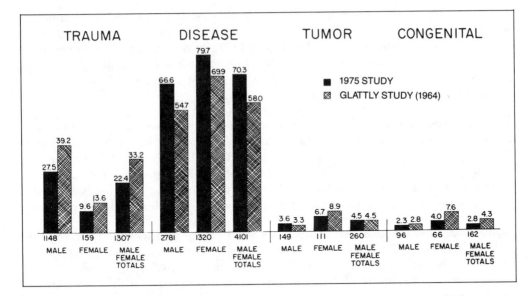

Figure 1–3. Distribution of amputees by cause and sex, comparing studies done in 1975 with 1964. (From Kay HW, Newman JD. Relative incidence of new amputations. *Orthot Prosthet* 1975; **29**:8, with permission.)

Trauma. In some accidents or trauma, part or all of the limb may be removed completely, or autoamputated, because of the accident; or the limb may be damaged to such an extent that removal of the limb may be required following the accident. Figure 1–3 from Kay and Newman[8] demonstrates a 22.4% trauma-related cause for amputation. Common accidental causes of traumatic amputation include the following: automobile accidents, farm machinery accidents, fire arms, freezing, electrical burns, and power-tool accidents. In some cases, as in severe brachial plexus injuries, damage to the nervous system results in paralysis to the limb that is debilitating enough to require amputation. These levels are said to be elective, since they are usually not life threatening and often may be performed at a level elected by the surgeon. Knowledge of prosthetic restoration is critical so as to elect the most functional level for the patient.

Disease. Vascular disease may lead to amputation. Diseases that may cause vascular or circulatory problems are diabetes, arterial sclerosis, and Buerger's disease. In these instances the blood supply to the limb is inadequate, so that necrosis or dry gangrene of the tissues occurs. In such cases it is usually the lower limb that is principally affected. Circulatory disorders are more common among elderly individuals, and thus the majority of amputations for vascular reasons occur in the lower limbs of these elderly persons. Kay and Newman[8] reported 70.3% of all new amputees to be of vascular disease origin. Furst and Humphrey[3] reported an 85% vascular or metabolic origin for 5,000 amputations annually in England and Wales. Of these 85%, men were two times as likely as women to need amputation, and overall 70% of all new amputees were 60 years of age or older. On another note, Furst and Humphrey[3] surveyed the wives of below-knee amputees to identify their perceptions of the commonest causes of amputation. Four of five wives felt that trauma was the leading cause and that the average age for amputation was 40 years less than it actually was. Often younger, nonvascular, below-knee amputees are the most visible amputees in our society. They are also a small minority of the entire amputee population. Infection is also a potential cause for amputation, although more recently, with the advent of more effective drugs, the number of amputations for this cause has been reduced.

Tumor. Amputation may also be undertaken as treatment for tumorous conditions. Primary bone tumors occur frequently in adolescents but can occur at any age. Figure 1–3 from Kay and Newman[8] shows that about 4.5% of all reported limb fittings are due to tumors. Figure 1–4 further demonstrates that 33.5% of these amputations occur between the ages of 11 and 20 years. Of further concern is the fact that bone tumors tend to occur more proximal in the limb, making high-level limb ablation necessary.

Congenital Amputations and Malformations. In some instances all or part of a limb is deficient at birth. These absences may be either the result of a congenital amputation or a limb deficiency or defect. Congenital amputations, although rare, connote the one-time presence of the limb and its amputation, in utero, often the result of a constriction band or ring. Limb deficiencies are malformations of the limb bud, occurring around day 28 in utero, yielding something less than a normal extremity. Although both may be treated in a similar manner prosthetically, limb deficiencies tend to require nonstandard prostheses and are often surgically converted to more standard anatomic and/or prosthetic levels. One such common condition is the congenital absence of the left forearm, the so-called terminal-transverse–congenital-limb deficiency of the forearm. Limb deficiencies, however, can occur anywhere and in any combination.

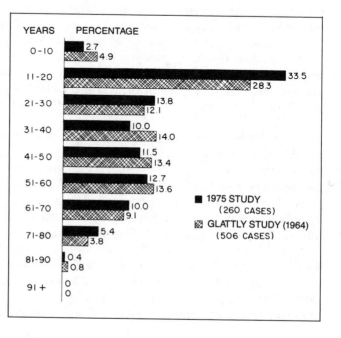

Figure 1–4. Occurrence of tumor-related amputation by age, comparing studies done in 1975 with 1964. (From Kay HW, Newman JD. Relative incidence of new amputations. *Orthot Prosthet* 1975; **29**:8, with permission.)

Reactions and Adjustments Associated With Amputation and Use of a Prosthesis

Amputation of a body segment results in problems that are physical, psychologic, social, and, possibly, economic in nature. These various problems are closely interrelated and often require simultaneous solutions, since one solution may affect other problems. Careful listening on the part of the health care professional may hasten the rehabilitation process or may prevent problems from ever occurring. Good, complete communications with the amputee and family are essential for adjustment to a new way of life or at least a different way of doing things.

Physical Factors. The most obvious problems associated with loss of a limb segment are the functional limitations that result. There is a primary satisfaction enjoyed by all individuals who are able to control their body and to perform a variety of desired activities. In addition to the satisfaction derived from the use of one's physical faculties, there are other satisfactions that are achieved only through the use of prehensile or ambulatory functions as intervening steps or prerequisites to other activities.

When the amputee approaches a physical task, the following alternatives are available: (1) avoid performing the task; (2) compensate for the lost segment by increased use of the remaining segments; or (3) perform the activity by using an artificial replacement for the missing segment. Depending on the particular task and the patient's level of amputation, any one or a combination of these alternatives may be used. In any event, at least some minor restrictions and limitations occur in accomplishing the activity so that total normal satisfaction is never achieved.

As a general rule, lower-extremity prostheses replace lost function more adequately than upper-extremity prostheses. In the lower extremity, varying amounts of difficulty will be manifest depending on the level of amputation, the adequacy of the prosthetic device, the patient's general condition, and the patient's motivation. Since upper-extremity functions tend to be inherently more varied and complex, upper extremity devices cannot be expected to provide "near normal" function. As with the lower-limb amputee, the loss of function in the upper extremity increases very rapidly with each more proximal level of amputation. In both the lower and upper extremity, occurrence of bilateral amputation poses a drastic increase in loss of function compared to unilateral amputation.

In addition to the loss of motor function resulting from amputation, the amputee is also deprived of important sensory information normally present with an intact limb. This lack of sensory feedback is important in the lower limb but is probably more important in the upper limb and is the major limiting factor in the effective use of artificial hands and hooks.

Because the artificial limb is attached to the stump over soft tissue, there is a false joint between the skeletal system and the prosthesis. This insecure attachment usually results in feelings of instability and uncertainty in the control of the prosthetic device. This phenomenon is particularly important for weight bearing in the lower extremity. A secondary consequence of this unstable attachment to the skeletal system is the feeling that the artificial limb is heavier than an intact limb, even though, in fact, it may be considerably lighter.

Because the socket may be fitted over tissues that are not normally weight-bearing tissues, a number of secondary physical problems may occur related to the socket fit. These problems include edema resulting from a socket that is too tight at the proximal end, pressure problems leading to atrophy of muscle and subcutaneous fat, osteoporosis as a result of reduced skeletal weight bearing, boney spurs, allergic reactions to the socket material, cysts, infections, reduced blood flow, and neuromata at the site of amputation.

In addition to the problem of heat buildup within the socket, the amputee may have a problem with central body-temperature regulation due to the loss of body mass and its related surface area. Because of the lost body segment, perspiration over the rest of the body tends to increase, further compounding skin problems.

A general problem experienced by amputees is the overall increase in fatigue associated with "normal" activities. This factor is particularly important in lower-extremity amputees, since it has been clearly shown that ambulation using a prosthetic device considerably increases the energy required for this activity. Since the amputee must expend more energy for ambulatory functions, he or she has less energy available for other activities. This additional energy requirement is likely to have an impact on the amputee's motivation and willingness to participate in such activities.

For the amputee, conscious attention must often be paid to functions that are carried on more or less automatically with an intact limb. In other words, many functions that are controlled subcortically with an intact neuromusculoskeletal system require cortical attention by the amputee. Such attention requires additional motivation by the amputee and also limits the attention that can be given to concurrent activities. This problem tends to be more important in upper-extremity functions in which the amputee must use vision as a substitute for normal sensory feedback in prehensile activities.

Another type of problem experienced by the prosthetic wearer is the general discomfort associated with wearing the prosthetic device. What is referred to as a comfortable prosthetic fit is, in reality, a fit that offers the minimum tolerable degree of discomfort for the amputee. Prosthetic devices are fitted over tissues that are performing atypical functions, primarily weight bearing in the lower extremities. Until these tissues become adjusted to these new functions, significant discomfort may be experienced by the amputee.

A physical problem associated with amputation for the majority of amputees is the presence of phantom sensations in the limb that has been removed. Phantom sensation is defined as a painless awareness of the "presence" of the amputated part and often includes a mild tingling sensation. Phantom sensation is frequently incomplete, and the segments felt most often are those with the greatest sensory representation in the cerebral cortex. The foot and hand are usually felt more than other parts of the limb, and the thumb and great toe are usually areas of high awareness. If phantom sensation is painful and disagreeable, it is referred to as phantom pain. Phantom pain may be constant or intermittent and may vary greatly in intensity.[9] The three most commonly described types of phantom pain are (1) postural cramping or a squeezing sensation, (2) burning sensation and, (3) sharp, shooting pain. A mixture of these three types of pain is felt by some patients. In time phantom pain tends to disappear for most amputees, but the presence of phantom sensation tends to remain indefinitely for many individuals.

Phantom sensation and pain are not present in individuals with congenital amputations or deficiencies. In instances of crushing injuries or among older amputees, phantom pain tends to remain longer and to pose a greater problem. Once phantom pain becomes a problem, treatment is quite difficult, and treatment successes are few. One report by Sherman[9] lists 43 individual treatments for phantom pain, from lobotomies to injection to re-exploration/reamputation. Most treatments were reviewed by one author as successful and by another as being unsuccessful.

Psychosocial Factors. For some individuals the psychologic and social problems associated with amputation are of greater consequence than the physical problems. Grief is considered to be the universal reaction resulting from the loss of a limb segment. The grief reaction follows a predictable course that can be divided into the immediate impact phase, the recall phase, and the reconstruction or psychologic rehabilitation phase. All grief reactions are not the same, and each amputee's reaction is dependent upon his or her basic personality type. An essential factor in the grief process is the acceptance of the limb loss and the realization that the loss is permanent. Denial of the importance of the handicap or limb loss is not an uncommon phenomenon. Anger is also a common manifestation of the grieving process, and this anger may be directed to anyone who attempts to help the individual accept his or her loss. Anger may also be directed at parents, whom the patient may blame for "giving them" diabetes or other vascular diseases.

The sense of loss is dependent upon the amputated part and its significance to the amputee. Feelings of increased dependence as a result of amputation present further complicating factors. Changes in behavior and evidence of depression are also common reactions to limb amputation. During the recall phase the patient learns to talk about the loss and, in some cases, to make light of his or her previous reactions. In the final reconstruction phase the amputee adjusts to a new self-image and beings to direct his or her energies toward more constructive and satisfying activities. Most amputees work through all three phases of the grieving process, although some individuals remain fixed in the first or second phase.

Because the amputee depends upon a mechanical prosthetic device, he or she must learn to live with the awareness that the device may fail at any time. The amputee must anticipate some instances when he or she will fall down during ambulation or fail in simple acts of prehension using a prosthetic device. These failures are sources of embarrassment for the individual and have significant psychologic and social implications, since most societies have a relatively negative attitude toward people who fail.

Loss of acceptance by one's peers is another psychosocial factor affecting amputees. Social prejudices against disabled individuals have been reflected in literature, such as those directed at Captain Hook, Long John Silver, and other devious characters. These attitudes toward amputees are ingrained at an early age and are changed only very slowly. Parents of young children who are fitted with "hook" terminal devices react negatively when first shown such devices.

The term cosmesis refers to the visual appearance of the prosthetic device. Cosmetic problems tend to be of greater importance for the upper-extremity amputee than for the lower-extremity amputee, since the lower extremity is more easily covered with clothing. Young children tend to be less conscious of appearances than adolescents or adults. Since our society places great importance on the quality, adequacy, and conformity of one's physical appearance, individuals not meeting society's standards often suffer loss of group acceptance. Along with feelings of group rejection, the amputee may develop problems of an interpersonal nature.

Since artificial limbs are, in essence, mechanical devices, they are subject to a variety of low-level sounds associated with their operation. These sounds draw attention to the amputee and, again, send a message to others that the amputee is unusual in some way.

Vocational and Economic Factors. The occurrence of a limb amputation may have significant impact on an individual's ability to earn a living. Unskilled or semiskilled laborers tend to rely more on their physical abilities for gainful employment. The employability of these individuals is particularly affected by amputation, and it is this group of individuals who are least able to adjust to skilled or managerial positions. For individuals whose duties are professional, managerial, or executive, the economic adjustments to amputation are less significant. The large majority of unemployed and marginally employable amputees comes from lower socioeconomic groups. Hence an important adjustment to be made by amputees in this group is the need to relearn vocational skills. This often entails a major change in lifestyle. State offices of vocational rehabilitation were designed to help just such individuals.

Individual Reactions. For any given individual amputee, it is impossible to make generalizations about the relative significance of the physical, psychosocial, and vocational and economic problems associated with amputation. In most cases effective treatment results in the reduction of the number of the amputee's problems but fails to completely irradicate any one of them. Likewise, during the amputee's lifetime, different problems will assume greater and lesser importance, depending upon other factors.

Prosthetic Preoperative Evaluation

Ideally the clinic team begins its work as soon as it is determined that an amputation is necessary. The preoperative evaluation of any patient attempts to both gain information and transmit information. The information gained helps in determining the nature and severity of any potential problems that may be encountered during the postoperative course. The preoperative evaluation also serves as a time when the prospective amputee may ask any questions that have been harbored during the process of making the decision to proceed with the amputation. Questions may arise as to components, cosmesis, or other concerns about perceptions, taboos, or media images, all of which are of concern to the patient and family.

Patient Expectations. Questions concerning the expectations of the patient are important. This information, when coupled with the diagnostic and other team input, assists the members of the clinic team in developing a reasonable and workable treatment plan. It is also important to ascertain how the impending amputation will affect the patient's lifestyle. In the process of collecting necessary information concerning the patient's future, it is often helpful to contact a significant other, whether this person is a family member or not, that is, another person in the patient's life in whom trust may be placed, both by the clinic team members and the patient. This significant other often plays a role in the decision-making process and may be invaluable in effecting a successful transition back into the home and/or work environment once discharge from the hospital or care facility occurs.

Many decisions made by the amputee about the future will involve his or her vocation or avocation. The degree of motivation that the amputee brings to the postoperative situation will help determine the goals to which the ultimate prosthetic fitting may lead. Additionally, the type or intensity of the patient's vocation may assist the clinic team in making decisions about the type and strength of the components of the prosthetic device.

It is very important to assure the patient at the preoperative meeting that all questions are important and that all will be answered. It is important to deal with the subject of pain and the sensations of the lost limb and to communicate the normal and usual nature of these feelings. One of the questions usually asked by the soon-to-be amputee is "when" all these things are going to happen. It is common for the patient and his or her significant other to begin to focus on the prosthesis and the events following the amputation. This allows the physical therapist or other team member to enumerate the events and goals associated with both the early and late prosthetic phases and to put them in their proper time sequence.

Physical Examination. Along with a thorough review of the medical record and discussions among the members of the clinic team, the physical examination occurs. The discussion with the attending surgeon should reveal the anticipated level of amputation and any potential medical problems that may lead to a less-than-optimal result.

Before the amputation the physical therapist needs to know the patient's abilities with whatever walking aides that have been used prior to surgery. If the patient is a good crutch user, teaching him or her to use a new gait in expectation of the amputation saves some time and gives the patient an idea of what to expect following surgery. If the patient is unaccustomed to using crutches or a walker, it is a good time to teach him or her while there are no pain or balance problems. Since balance may be affected in the early postoperative days, balance routines may be demonstrated to educate the patient about what to expect following surgery. This is also a good time for the physical therapist to establish a helping rapport with the amputee and to demonstrate how future goals will be addressed together.

As a part of the overall preoperative evaluation, it is important to evaluate the strength and range of motion of both the involved and uninvolved limbs and joints. Normal prosthetic ambulation requires good range of motion and strength on both sides. The presence of fixed deformities limits the expectations for the patient but also assists in setting realistic goals. Accurate evaluation of proximal joint strength allows early exercise programs to target these areas, preparing them for later use.

It is not uncommon for patients to develop flexion contractures in the early postoperative days following amputation. It is therefore necessary to know that the contracture was not present prior to surgery and that it may be quickly dealt with and remedied. In cases of extreme flexion contractures, the patient should be given information concerning the nonstandard nature of the finished prosthesis. Often the managing surgeon will delay the elective procedure until all conservative measures of managing the contracture have been exhausted or until sound medical evidence indicates that a life-threatening situation exists.

AN OVERVIEW OF ORTHOTICS

Orthotics Users

The 3% of the American population who may benefit from application of an orthotic device include individuals who have been affected by a wide spectrum of neuromusculoskeletal diseases, trauma, and congenital problems. Although pediatric and geriatric applications are somewhat more prevalent, orthosis wearers include all age groups. Orthotic applications for specific problems will be discussed in Chapters 7, 9, and 11.

Orthotics Nomenclature

Just as in prosthetics, as various orthotic devices have been developed there has been a tendency to name them after the developer. This is especially true in regard to spinal orthotics. The need for a standardized nomenclature had been recognized for many years, but it was not until the 1960s that a joint effort to develop it was undertaken by the American Academy of Orthopaedic Surgeons, the Committee on Prosthetics-Orthotics Education of the National Academy of Sciences, and the American Orthotics and Prosthetics Association. A series of workshops resulted in the development of a nomenclature and its attendant terminology for orthotic devices and systems that has

TABLE 1–2. ORTHOTICS NOMENCLATURE

Upper-Limb Orthoses			
HO	hand orthosis		
WO	wrist orthosis	WHO	wrist-hand orthosis
EO	elbow orthosis	EWHO	elbow-wrist-hand orthosis
SO	shoulder orthosis	SEWHO	shoulder-elbow-wrist-hand orthosis
Spinal Orthoses			
CO	cervical orthosis	CTLSO	cervical-thoracic-lumbosacral orthosis
TO	thoracic orthosis	TLSO	thoracic-lumbosacral orthosis
LO	lumbar orthosis	LSO	lumbosacral orthosis
		SIO	sacroiliac orthosis
Lower-Limb Orthoses			
FO	foot orthosis	AFO	ankle-foot orthosis
KO	knee orthosis	KAFO	knee-ankle-foot orthosis
HO	hip orthosis	HKAFO	hip-knee-ankle-foot orthosis

become accepted in many parts of the world. The core of these descriptions are acronyms based on the major joints that an orthosis is intended to control or affect. For example, an ankle-foot orthosis is referred to as an AFO, and an orthosis that extends from the foot to the thigh is referred to as a knee-ankle-foot orthosis, or KAFO. Table 1–2 presents a summary of this nomenclature.

Reactions and Adjustments to Orthotics Use

The reactions and adjustments to wearing and depending on an orthotic device are similar to but often less dramatic than those associated with amputation and using a prosthesis. They are, nonetheless, important factors that must be taken seriously and dealt with conscientiously.

REFERENCES

1. *National Health Survey. Use of Special Aids-1969.* Rockville, Md: US Dept. of Health, Education, and Welfare publication; 1969. HSM 73–1504.
2. *National Health Survey. Use of Special Aids—1977.* Rockville, Md: National Center for Health Statistics; 1974. US Dept. of Health, Education, and Welfare publication, 126, series 10.
3. Furst L, Humphrey M. Coping with the loss of a leg. *Prosthet Orthot Int* 1983; 7:152–156.
4. Practitioner Level Programs. *Orthot Prosthet* 1984; **38**(2); 20–68.
5. *Ponte Vedra II: Orthotic/Prosthetic Future.* Washington, DC: American Orthotic and Prosthetic Association, 1976.
6. Shurr DG. The delivery of orthotic and prosthetic services in America—a physical therapist's view. *Orthot Prosthet* 1984; **38**(1):55–63.
7. Nickel V. Orthotics in America. *Clin Ortho* 1974; **102**:10–17.
8. Kay HW, Newman JD. Relative incidences of new amputations. *Orthot Prosthet* 1975; **29**(2): 3–16.
9. Sherman RA. Limb pain and stump blood circulation. *Orthopaedics* 1984; **7**(8):1319–1320.

CHAPTER 2

Methods, Materials, and Mechanics

This chapter presents an overview of the processes and materials used to produce prosthetic and orthotic devices. Also presented are some common biomechanical considerations that must be taken into account when making and applying these devices. Although there are some factors that are specific to either prosthetics or orthotics, there are, by far, many more commonalities than differences in the methods and materials used to produce these devices. Therefore this chapter will focus on methods, materials, and mechanical concepts that apply to both prosthetics and orthotics.

FABRICATION METHODS

Steps in the Provision of a Prosthesis/Orthosis

The delivery of any prosthetic or orthotic device, from a simple finger splint to a complex lower-limb prosthesis, should include the six steps outlined in Table 2–1. As was briefly discussed in Chapter 1, the prescription specifying the type of device to be delivered should, ideally, be the result of consultations among the members of a multidisciplinary clinic team and should be based on a thorough evaluation of the patient's needs and functional goals.

Once a decision has been reached about the device to be used, the prosthetist/orthotist then proceeds to take the measurements and/or impressions needed to produce, or at least select, the device. Measurements are likely to include such items as the lengths and circumferences of body segments, locations of bony landmarks and tendons, joint ranges of motion, and strength. Careful attention is also paid to other factors such as the presence of scar tissue, neuromas, edema, and weight problems.[1] When a prosthesis or custom-molded orthosis has been prescribed, the measurement process includes taking an impression of the body segment (or residual limb in the case of a prosthesis). This impression taking is usually achieved by taking a plaster cast of the segment, making sure that the plaster is in close contact with the limb segment at

TABLE 2–1. STEPS IN PROVIDING A PROSTHESIS/ORTHOSIS

Step 1	evaluation/prescription
Step 2	measurement/impression taking (casting)
Step 3	fabrication/bench alignment
Step 4	fitting/static alignment
Step 5	modification/dynamic alignment
Step 6	re-evaluation/follow-up

specific anatomic sites that will be important to the function of the completed device. Figures 2–1A and 2–2A illustrate impression taking using plaster casts.

The third step in the provision of an orthotic or prosthetic device is the actual fabrication. In the simplest case this step may consist of merely selecting the proper size of a prefabricated off-the-shelf device, with only minor adjustments based on the measurements taken from the patient. More commonly, in the case of a custom-made device, the prosthetist/orthotist uses the measurements and plaster cast to produce a positive model of the body segment to which the device will be fitted. Figures 2–1B and 2–2B illustrate this step in the process. The positive model is not simply an exact duplicate of the body segment but is skillfully modified by the prosthetist/orthotist so that the final device will have specific areas of increased contact (pressure) and other areas of reduced contact (pressure). If the device being fabricated is a lower-limb prosthesis, the prosthetist will initially arrange or "align" the foot and other components of the device using established guidelines referred to as "bench alignment," which will be discussed in Chapters 4 and 5.

Once the device has been fabricated, the next step is fitting it to the patient, that is, trying it on to see how it fits and feels. At this stage attention is paid to whether the forces and pressures applied by the device are in the desired locations and of magnitudes that the patient can tolerate. If the device is a lower-limb prosthesis, this fitting step includes an assessment of whether the foot and other components of the device are adequately aligned for standing and weight bearing.

The fifth step in the provision of an orthosis or prosthesis is to modify or to fine tune the device after the patient has tried to function with it. This step may include relatively minor adjustments such as the addition of padding or the grinding or trimming of material. It might also consist of more major changes such as the substitution of different components or refabrication of part of the device. In the case of lower-limb prosthetics, and to some extent orthotics, this step includes the process of dynamic alignment wherein fine adjustments are made to the device to achieve the patient's optimal gait pattern.

The final but equally important step in providing a device is re-evaluation and follow-up by the clinic team to determine that the patient's needs continue to be met by the device. Not only may the device function differently due to wear and tear but the patient's status may fluctuate due to changes in functional ability, lifestyle, body weight and proportions, and similar factors.

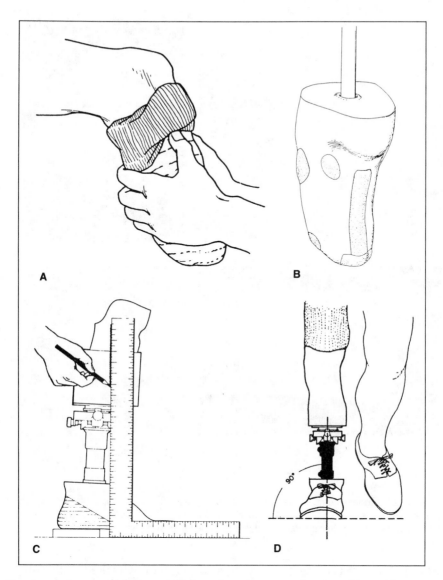

Figure 2–1. Prosthetics fabrication techniques: (**A**) impression taking using a plaster cast; (**B**) modified positive plaster model of residual limb; (**C**) bench aligning a below-knee prosthetic limb; (**D**) dynamic alignment.

Fabrication Options

There are several different options and terms regarding fabrication of prosthetic and orthotic devices that need to be understood. The distinction between off-the-shelf and custom fabrication has already been mentioned in the previous section. In concept,

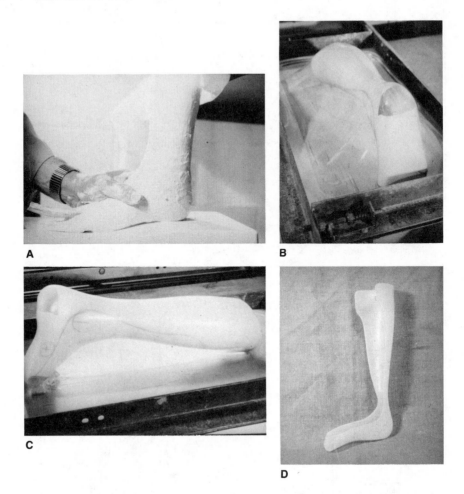

Figure 2–2. Orthotics fabrication techniques: (**A**) impression taking using a plaster cast; (**B**) heated plastic sheet being vacuum formed over a postive plaster model of the limb segment; (**C**) trimlines showing through cooled plastic; (**D**) finished plastic-molded AFO.

devices and components that are mass produced and stocked by the prosthetist/orthotist are likely to be of a more consistent quality, to be less expensive, and to be delivered faster to the patient than devices and components that are individually manufactured one at a time. Similarly, standardized, interchangeable, off-the-shelf components should make replacement and repair of devices easier and faster. For these reasons there has been a clear trend in prosthetics and orthotics to use as many premanufactured modular components and devices as possible. In many cases, however, a portion of the device (and sometimes the entire device) must be custom made to properly fit the patient and to accomplish the intended goals. Precise impression taking (casting) is, and will likely continue to be, an integral part of the delivery of most prosthetic and orthotics devices.

Another important distinction in regard to fabricating prosthetic and orthotic devices is between local and central fabrication. Costs associated with certified personnel, plastics, ovens, vacuum forming, and Occupational Safety and Health Administration regulations in the late 1960s and early 1970s encouraged the development of central fabrication, or production of devices from a centralized geographic location separate from the site where measurement, delivery, and fitting of the devices occur. Central fabrication allows complex and expensive technology to be used without the need for each facility to purchase, use, and maintain expensive, modern, high-technology equipment. Other advantages of central fabrication include better use of the certified practitioner's time, making it possible for him or her to serve more patients and for the prosthetist/orthotist to have a more professional location, apart from the smell, dust, and congestion of a fabrication site. Some disadvantages of central fabrication include increased chances for communication problems with the technicians who actually make the devices, particularly with nonstandard applications, and possible additional time delays for shipping models and finished devices. Central fabrication is a natural extension of prefabrication. If an entire device needs custom fabrication, it can be fabricated at a centralized location from a cast taken by the certified practitioner and sent to the laboratory. This system is analogous to the current production of dentures, eyeglasses, and other medical or dental devices. In the future, central fabrication will allow the practitioner to continue to survive economically, as profit margins are held in check by governmental controls of health care costs.

Specifications for the "Ideal" Prosthesis/Orthosis

In producing a prosthetic/orthotic device, there are certain "ideal" design specifications that are kept in mind, but rarely all are achieved. Table 2–2 lists some of these specifications. Foremost among these specifications is the desire to have the device function as intended. The device should be simple in design, easy for the patient to learn to use, and the device should continue to function dependably with little need for repair or replacement. Also of great importance to the use of the device is the comfort of the fit. If the device causes areas of high skin pressure, irritation, or reaction, it is unlikely that the patient will continue to use it. Likewise, the device should be easy to put on (don) and to take off (doff) and should be lightweight and somewhat adjustable to accommodate minor fluctuations in the patient's size.

Cosmesis, or the appearance, smell, and sound of the device, is also important. As mentioned in the previous chapter, many individuals in our society are hesitant to draw attention to themselves by appearing, smelling, or making sounds that are "abnormal" or unusual. Some devices may provide good function but may go unused because of

TABLE 2–2. SPECIFICATIONS FOR THE "IDEAL" PROSTHESIS/ORTHOSIS

Function	meets user's needs, simple, easily learned, dependable
Comfort	fits well, easy to put on and take off, lightweight, adjustable
Cosmesis	looks, smells, sounds "normal," easily cleaned, stain resistant
Fabrication	fast, modular, readily and widely available
Economics	affordable, worth cost

these factors. Because they are often in constant contact with body tissues, most prosthetic and orthotic devices need to be stain resistant and easy to clean.

Ideally prostheses and orthoses are fabricated and delivered quickly; use a maximum number of prefabricated, modular components; and are widely and readily available to those who need them. Similarly, the ideal is for these devices to be affordable by those in need and worth the cost for the improved function they provide.

MATERIALS

Material Characteristics Important in Prosthetics and Orthotics

There are several characteristics of materials that determine their suitability for use in prosthetics and orthotics. Table 2–3 lists the most important of these characteristics.

Certainly strength, or the maximum external load that a material can sustain, is important, especially in lower-limb and spinal applications where force levels may be quite high. An equally important material characteristic that must be taken into account is stiffness. This characteristic defines the amount of bending or compression (strain) that occurs in response to the amount of load (stress) applied. In some applications, such as lower-limb prosthetics and orthotics, there is a need for materials that are very stiff and rigid and that allow virtually no flexion or bending when loaded. In other components of the same device, however, it may be highly desirable to use very flexible materials to conform to changing body segments, to absorb shock, and to store "elastic" energy. Both the strength and stiffness of a given component of a prosthetic or orthotic device depend not only on the material used in that component but also on the thickness and shape of the material. Cylindrical and semicircular shapes and components with ridges, flanges, or corrugations are inherently stronger and stiffer than flat, thin sections of material.

Durability, or fatigue resistance, refers to the ability of a material to withstand repeated loading and unloading cycles. In nearly all materials, repeated loading reduces the maximum strength and causes failure or fracture at a load level lower than that which occurs before the material is fatigued. Since orthotic and prosthetic devices may be loaded hundreds of thousands and sometimes millions of cycles,[2] fatigue resistance is an important characteristic. Areas of particular concern in regard to fatigue or failure occur at any interface between two materials that have significantly different properties, such as plastic and metal. Some materials are also especially prone to failure at sites where the surface has been scratched or "notched."

TABLE 2–3. IMPORTANT CHARACTERISTICS OF PROSTHETIC AND ORTHOTICS MATERIALS

Strength	the maximum external load that can be withstood
Stiffness	the stress/strain or force-to-displacement ratio
Durability (fatigue resistance)	the ability to withstand repeated loading
Density	the weight per unit volume
Corrosion resistance	resistance to chemical degradation
Ease of fabrication	equipment and techniques needed to shape it

Density, or weight per unit volume, is a continual concern in selecting materials for prosthetics and orthotics. Nearly always the goal is to make the device as lightweight as possible to minimize the energy required to support and move it possibly hundreds or thousands of times each day.

Two additional material characteristics that need to be considered are corrosion resistance and ease of fabrication. Limitations due to either one of these factors can severely limit the applicability of a particular material to prosthetic and orthotic devices. Ease of fabrication is especially important in custom-molded applications, since materials must be readily transformed into a soft, malleable state to conform to a model of a body segment. There are many "space-age" materials with several desirable characteristics, except for the fact that they are not easily formed, shaped, or tooled for prosthetic and orthotic applications.

A final practical consideration that affects the selection of which materials get used in prosthetic and orthotic devices is cost and availability. Ideal materials are readily available at reasonable costs. Clearly, no one material has the required characteristics for all applications or, as may be the case, the required characteristics for all the different components of a single device.[3]

Classes of Materials

Based on consideration of the material characteristics discussed above, several classes of materials are commonly used in prosthetics and orthotics. These materials are listed in Table 2–4.

Wood. Wood (principally maple and hickory) is used commonly as the major component in prosthetic feet. Basswood, willow, poplar, and linden wood are often used for prosthetic knees and shins.[1] These wooden components are lightweight, strong, inexpensive, easily shaped, and consistent in texture. Use of wood in orthotic systems is rare.

Leather. Leather is a material that has traditionally been, and continues to be, in common use in both prosthetics and orthotics. Leather (principally vegetable-tanned

TABLE 2–4. CLASSES OF MATERIALS COMMONLY USED IN PROSTHETICS AND ORTHOTICS

Wood
Leather
Fabric
Rubber
Metal
  Steel
  Aluminum
  Titanium and magnesium
Plastics
  Thermoplastics
  Thermosets

cowhide) is used for suspension straps, waist belts, socket liners, and protective coverings (fairings) over knee and hip joints in prosthetics. In addition to its superior use in the construction of footwear, leather is also used for molded arch supports, cuffs, straps, laces, linings, and coverings for orthoses.

Fabric. Fabrics used in prosthetic and orthotic devices may be made of wool, cotton, silk, or a number of synthetic materials such as nylon, olefin, polyester, rayon, or vinyl. These materials may be woven or knitted, although some may be molded with pressure, heat, or chemicals. Whenever a fabric must be fitted to a complex, three-dimensional shape, knitting is usually the preferred technique.[3] In prosthetic applications, fabrics are used for waist belts, straps, harnesses, and, most prevalently, for prosthetics socks, which function similarly to athletic socks, keeping the skin dry, cushioning the limb, and taking up space to improve the fit of the prosthesis on the limb segment. Prosthetic socks are commonly made of wool, cotton, or blends of these with nylon or other synthetic materials.[1] In orthotic applications, fabrics are used primarily for fastening or for less rigid supports, such as in corsets, belts, and stockings.[3]

Rubber. The elastic properties and high friction coefficient of rubber materials make them useful for padding in prosthetic and orthotic devices, for seals in hydraulic and pneumatic mechanisms, and for heels and bumpers in prosthetic feet and special footwear.

Metal. The three types of metals most appropriate for use in prosthetics and orthotics are steel, aluminum, and alloys of titanium and magnesium. The major properties that affect their usefulness are their maximum strength, stiffness, and weight per unit volume (density). Figure 2–3 shows a comparison of these three properties.

   Steel, including corrosion-resistant stainless steel, has the advantages of low cost, availability, and relative ease of fabrication. It is strong, rigid, and fatigue resistant, but, unfortunately, it is also relatively heavy. Steel is widely found in prefabricated prosthetic and orthotic joints, metal bands, cuffs, cables, springs, bearings, and hydraulic and pneumatic components.

   Aluminum is a much lighter metal than steel with a high strength-to-weight ratio and is particularly useful in upper-extremity, pediatric, and other applications where weight is a major consideration. The primary disadvantage of aluminum is its relatively poor resistance to fatigue at high-load levels or at high rates of repeated loading.

   Titanium and magnesium alloys have strengths comparable to steel but are substantially lighter in weight with good corrosion resistance. Their principal disadvantage is their limited availability and relative high cost.[3]

Plastics. The increased availability and use of plastic materials has had a dramatic impact on prosthetics and orthotics in recent years. The term plastic can refer to any synthetic material that can be molded, extruded, laminated, or hardened into any form.[3] Some major advantages in using these plastic materials is that they are lightweight, many can be readily formed into complex anatomic shapes, they tend to be nontoxic,

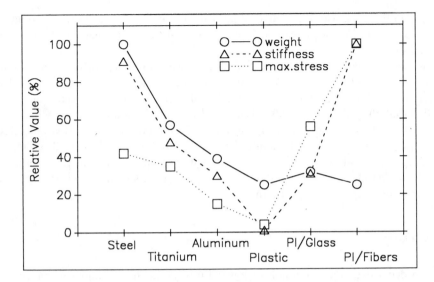

Figure 2–3. Comparison of weight, stiffness, and maximum stress of materials commonly employed in prosthetic and orthotic devices. (Adapted from Henshaw J. The design of the orthotic appliance. In: Murphy G, ed. *The Advance in Orthotics. Baltimore, Md*: Williams and Wilkins; 1976:146.)

and they are generally impervious to body fluids. In prosthetics and orthotics, a distinction can be made between two major types of plastics, thermoplastics and thermosetting plastics.

Thermoplastics are materials that become soft and malleable when heated and then become hard again when cooled. Their potential uses in prosthetics and orthotics in the United States were first realized in the late 1960s. In the heated state they can be molded and remolded repeatedly. Thermoplastic materials that become workable below 80°C (180°F) are generally referred to as low-temperature thermoplastics and, with care, can usually be formed directly on a body segment.[4] This type of material is most useful for upper-limb orthotic applications and for temporary use such as in fracture braces, since they usually have limited strength and fatigue resistance. High-temperature thermoplastics (malleable above 80°C or 180°F) must be shaped over a model and include materials such as acrylic, polyethylene, polypropylene, polycarbonate, ABS, PVC, and others. They are usually used in the fabrication of permanent prosthetic and orthotic devices using vacuum-forming methods. There are also a number of soft-foam interface plastics such as pelite, plastizote, and aliplast, which are used principally as liners or padding.[5]

In contrast to thermoplastics, thermosetting materials develop a permanent shape when formed and cannot be reheated and reformed. Because of the heat they give off during curing, thermosetting plastics, principally polyester resins, must be formed over a model. They are usually laminated with layers of natural or synthetic cloth and can be sanded, ground down, drilled, and riveted. They also can be pigmented in an attempt to match a patient's skin color. As can be seen from Figure 2–3, the addition of glass or fiber elements to plastic material dramatically increases its maximum strength and stiffness. The majority of prosthetic limbs produced today are made of thermosetting plastic laminates.

The uses of plastics in the construction of prostheses and orthoses are evolving quickly. In a recent survey,[6] 17% of the responding practitioners indicated that their patients in need of leg orthoses received 100% plastic devices. Sixty-one percent indicated that they delivered 75% plastic and only 25% metal devices, whereas only 15% used less than 25% plastic and, therefore, 75% metal orthoses. Reasons cited for using plastic instead of metal included weight, cosmesis, and versatility. Of those responding, the most commonly cited disadvantage of plastic was in the use of ankle-foot orthosis (AFO), where the inability to adjust the ankle in dorsiflexion or plantar flexion was often cited as a problem.

MECHANICS

Before proceeding to a discussion of lower-limb biomechanics and specific prosthetic and orthotic devices in subsequent chapters, it is important that consideration be given to three general (bio)mechanical topics that are applicable to nearly all prosthetic and/or orthotic devices.

Moments and Force Couples

When an orthosis is attached to a body segment, it is intended to exert a force on that segment to limit or to control an abnormal or unwanted motion. Although some component of the applied force may be directed along the axis of the segment, a significant rotational component is almost always present, tending to affect rotation of the anatomic joint. This rotational interaction of an orthotic device with body segments always involves what is referred to as a three-point force system or, sometimes, a three-point pressure system. Rotational forces or moments are not possible unless there are at least three points of contact between the device and the limb segment(s). Figure 2–4 illustrates some examples of three-point force systems.

In contrast to an orthosis, which is a device designed to apply forces and moments to body segments, amputees are usually involved in using their remaining limb segments to apply forces and moments to an external device, their prosthesis. In applying moments to move or to prevent motion of a prosthesis, a force couple must be exerted on the prosthesis. This force couple usually has a distal component in the direction of the intended moment and a proximal component that is in the opposite direction. Figure 2–5 illustrates common sites of force application in lower limb prosthetics.

In both prosthetic and orthotic applications, it is desirable to use the longest possible lever arms when applying moments to or from a device. A longer lever arm means that the same moment can be generated with a smaller force, since the moment is equal to the product of the force and the lever arm. Reducing forces is the principal means of minimizing pressures on body tissues.

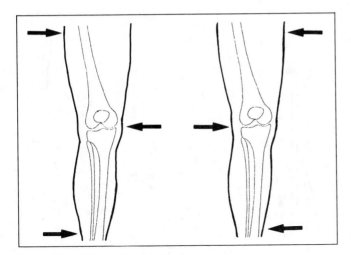

Figure 2–4. Example of a three-point force system used in knee orthotics.

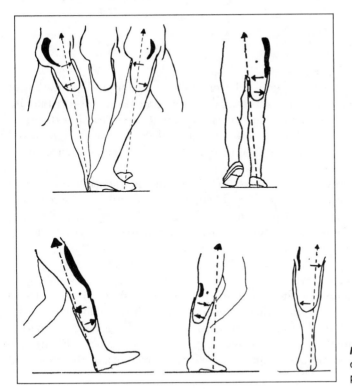

Figure 2–5. Examples of force-couple application in lower-limb prosthetics.

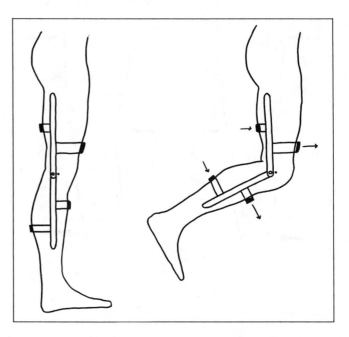

Figure 2–6. Example of malalignment between an anatomic and orthotic joint axis.

Pressure Tolerance of Tissues

Different biological tissues have markedly different tolerances for the application of external pressure. Anatomic sites with substantial muscle and fat tissue can tolerate higher pressures than bony prominences and areas containing superficial blood vessels and nerves. Contouring and padding to use pressure-tolerant areas and to avoid pressure-intolerant areas is an important element in the skillful fabrication of most prosthetic and orthotic devices.

Pressure is defined as force per unit area. Besides reducing the applied force (by maximizing lever arms), the other strategy for reducing tissue pressure is to increase the area over which the force is applied. This is an important consideration when decisions are made regarding the location and size of the bands or cuffs of an orthosis or regarding the length at which a limb segment should be amputated.

Alignment of Joint Axes

Alignment between the anatomic joint axis and the orthotic (and sometimes prosthetic) joint axis can be very important. If, intentionally or accidently, the axes do not coincide, additional sets of forces are likely to occur at various locations during the range of movement. These forces may include both compression and shearing.[7,8] Figure 2–6 illustrates some possible effects of malalignment between an orthotic and anatomic joint axis.

REFERENCES

1. Quigley M. Prosthetic methods and materials. In: *Atlas of Limb Prosthetics*. St. Louis, Mo: Mosby; 1981.
2. Henshaw J. The design of the orthotic appliance. In: Murphy G, ed. *The Advance in Orthotics*. Baltimore, Md: Williams & Wilkins; 1976.
3. Redford J, Licht S. Materials for orthotics. In: Redford, J, ed. *Orthotics Etcetera*. Baltimore, Md: Williams & Wilkins; 1986.
4. Compton J, Edlestein J. New plastics for forming directly on the patient. *Prosthet Orthot Int* 1978; **2**:43.
5. Showers D, Strunck M. Sheet plastics and their applications in orthotics and prosthetics. *Orthot Prosthet* 1985; **38**(4):41–48.
6. Pritham C. Analysis of the results from the questionnaire on metal vs. plastic orthoses. *Clin Prosthet Orthot* 1983; **7**(3):4.
7. Condie D. The mechanics of lower limb bracing. In: Murphy G, ed. *The Advance in Orthotics*. Baltimore, Md: Williams & Wilkins; 1976.
8. Smith E, Juvinall R. Mechanics of orthotics. In: Redford J, ed. *Orthotics Etcetera*. ed. Baltimore, Md: Williams & Wilkins; 1986.

CHAPTER 3

Biomechanics of the Lower Limb

Because of its special role in weight bearing and mobility, orthotic and prosthetic devices for the lower extremity must be based on a sound understanding of lower-limb biomechanics. This chapter considers the biomechanical functions of the lower limb especially as they relate to human ambulation. It is not intended as a comprehensive treatise on human gait but as a review of those functions that compose "normal" gait and of the factors to be considered when trying to restore or substitute for normal functioning by means of an orthotic or prosthetic device. The discussion will not include ambulation on stairs, ramps, and side slopes nor will it include the use of assistive devices.

FUNCTIONAL ROLE OF THE LOWER EXTREMITIES

The primary function of the lower extremities is to provide mobility, a means of travel from one place to another to see, to hear, to perform manual tasks, to participate in the whole range of human activities. While continuously opposing the force of gravity, the lower limbs must provide controlling and supporting forces during starting, stopping, and movement on level and uneven surfaces as well as during the transitions to and from the seated and lying positions. Safe and efficient accomplishment of all these tasks requires a neuromusculoskeletal system that is structurally sound, highly articulated, capable of a wide range of force development, and regulated by a sensitive, adaptable, control system. Because of inherent differences in body proportions, level of coordination, motivation, and similar factors, each individual's movement pattern is unique. Yet because everyone is subject to the same physical principles and because everyone has the same basic anatomic and physiologic makeup, normal human movements are accomplished in very much the same way by most healthy individuals.

Stauffer et al[1] have categorized ambulators into four classes. Class I includes those individuals who are nonambulatory. They cannot stand or walk but use a wheelchair for getting around. Class II individuals are considered exercise ambulators. They are able to stand and take a few steps with the aid of orthoses and/or assistive devices but use walking principally as part of a therapy session at home, in school, or in the hospital. Stauffer's third classification is household ambulator. These individuals are able to walk independently about the house but often use a wheelchair when out of the house. The fourth classification is community ambulator. These individuals walk most of the time, both indoors and outdoors, using a wheelchair rarely. This functional classification scheme can be very useful in describing patient performance and in goal setting.

When one or more components of the lower limb mobility system is altered or absent because of pathological, traumatic, or congenital factors, external devices may be provided in an attempt to maximize the individual's functional abilities. To understand the prosthetic and orthotic components that are intended to substitute for normal abilities, the major factors related to lower-extremity mobility must be understood. Walking represents the most common dynamic functional activity.

THE GAIT CYCLE

The sequential repetition of (approximately) the same movements of the major joints of the body during ambulation is referred to as the gait cycle. Figure 3–1 presents some of the terminology that is used to describe the foot contact events that occur during normal gait and to differentiate the various periods or phases that occur. The gait of healthy individuals is characterized by near symmetry in the temporal and distance aspects of foot contact with the supporting surface. Although achieving a normal foot contact pattern is a worthwhile general treatment objective, this goal cannot realistically be met by patients whose locomotor system is substantially different from normal as the result of disease, trauma, or congenital abnormality. A compromise is usually reached that includes such factors as gait efficiency, safety, comfort, and cosmesis. Often the symmetry of gait is abandoned as the individual attempts to compensate for a unilateral sensorimotor deficiency.

WALKING SPEED

Energy cost studies have indicated that for normal individuals a symmetric gait of approximately 1.3 m/sec (or approximately 80 m/min) is an optimal method and speed of walking. However, a wide range of available "free" speeds exists among healthy individuals depending on the location of and motivation for the activity. An individual's self-selected, or free, walking speed also tends to vary directly with height and somewhat inversely with age, although the influence of these two factors is highly variable.

When there is a neural, muscular, or skeletal deficit, the walking speed that may be optimal from an energy-cost viewpoint is often compromised for the sake of greater stability, less pain, and/or an enhanced feeling of security. This compromise is almost always exhibited as a decrease in walking speed. In general, slower walking speeds require reduced ranges of joint motion and slower movements as well as reduced forces and reduced rates of change of forces. To slow down is the most common general

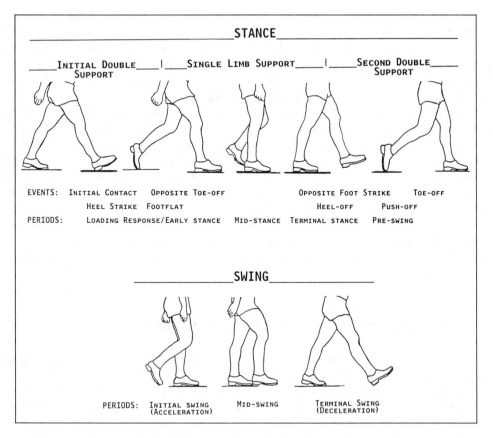

STANCE

____INITIAL DOUBLE____|____SINGLE LIMB SUPPORT____|____SECOND DOUBLE____
         SUPPORT   SUPPORT

EVENTS: INITIAL CONTACT   OPPOSITE TOE-OFF   OPPOSITE FOOT STRIKE   TOE-OFF
         HEEL STRIKE   FOOTFLAT   HEEL-OFF   PUSH-OFF
PERIODS: LOADING RESPONSE/EARLY STANCE   MID-STANCE   TERMINAL STANCE   PRE-SWING

SWING

PERIODS: INITIAL SWING   MID-SWING   TERMINAL SWING
           (ACCELERATION)   (DECELERATION)

Figure 3–1. Terms used to describe the phases, periods, and events during human locomotion.

strategy used by patients to cope with locomotor deficits and is generally related to the severity of impairment.

ENERGETICS OF GAIT

The major consequence of a slow and/or asymmetric gait is reduced efficiency, that is, increased energy expenditure for each meter walked. In normal gait the body's center of gravity (located just anterior to the second sacral vertebra) progresses smoothly on a nearly sinusoidal path throughout the gait cycle. The movement of the center of gravity is the result of all the summated forces and motions of the major joints of the body. The center of gravity moves in three dimensions, with a speedup and slowdown, a vertical rise and fall with each step, and a lateral cycle of motion during each stride. The general rule is that the smoother the path of the center of gravity, the less energy expended by the walker. Unnecessary, increased, or abrupt movements of the body's center of gravity during gait are the result of less-than-optimal joint motions and less-than-optimal use of muscle power. Each time the center of gravity goes down, it must be raised. Each time there is an exaggerated lateral movement, muscular energy must be expended to restore the system. Each time there is an abrupt decrease in forward speed, muscle power must be used to regain forward progression.

To traverse the same distance at the same speed with an altered movement pattern will require a greater rate of energy expenditure and a greater energy expenditure for each meter traveled. If an individual cannot or is not willing to increase the rate of energy expenditure, he or she may choose to walk more slowly. This strategy will decrease the energy expenditure rate, but because of the prolonged time in transit, the energy used per meter will be further increased. Most individuals with a locomotor deficit arrive at a compromise between the rate of energy expenditure and energy efficiency. This compromise is usually reflected in their "preferred" walking speed. Figure 3–2 shows examples of energy expenditure and energy efficiency at various walking speeds in healthy subjects and in individuals requiring orthotic and prosthetic devices.

LOWER LIMB FUNCTIONS DURING AMBULATION

A detailed examination of the normal kinematics and kinetics of the major joints of the lower limbs during ambulation is beyond the focus of this presentation, but a graphic summary of important factors is presented in Figure 3–3. Also represented in Figure 3–3 is the activity of the major muscle groups normally responsible for producing and controlling these movements.

Of direct relevance to orthotic and prosthetic applications is a consideration of the functions that are provided as a result of these controlled motions. With a sound understanding of normal gait functions, the clinician is in a position to intelligently select and provide devices to substitute for those functions.

The following sections will consider the major gait functions provided by the foot-ankle, knee, and hip along with a general presentation of some devices and strategies commonly used to externally augment or substitute for those functions. More detailed descriptions of specific components and devices are presented in later chapters.

Foot-Ankle Functions During Gait

From a gait-function point of view, five gait functions of the foot-ankle can be identified.

Surface Adaptation. The first foot-ankle gait function to be considered occurs in the frontal plane and is the ability of the foot-ankle to adapt to uneven surfaces (Fig. 3–4). This is a very important function when walking on other than smooth, flat, straight surfaces. Normally the mobility of the subtalar and other joints allows the foot to be placed and maintained in a variety of attitudes throughout the stance phase of gait. Because it requires such intricate and variable muscular control, surface adaptation is a

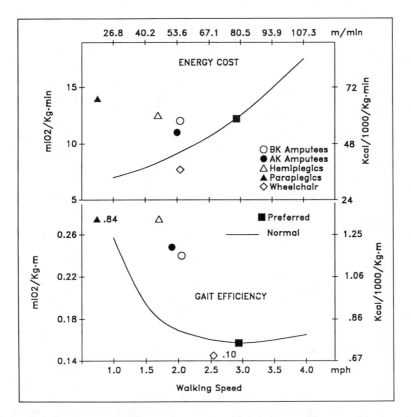

Figure 3–2. Energy cost (milliliters of oxygen or kilocalories per kilogram of body weight each minute) and gait efficiency (milliliters of oxygen or kilocalories per kilogram of body weight for each meter walked) for normal, "healthy" individuals (solid line) and for groups of individuals having amputations, hemiplegia, paraplegia, or using a wheelchair for mobility. The solid square represents the "preferred" walking speed for normal subjects (BK = below-knee; AK = above-knee).

foot-ankle function that is very difficult to substitute for or provide externally. With only a few exceptions, this function is usually sacrificed in lower-limb orthotic and prosthetic devices.

Shock Absorption. Immediately following the initial contact of the foot with the floor until the foot is flat, the foot-ankle normally assists in absorbing the "shock" of the body weight being loaded on the limb or, more specifically, in decreasing the rate of rise of the ground reaction force. Normally 15 or so degrees of controlled plantar flexion of the ankle is regulated by the eccentric contraction of the dorsiflexor musculature. Uncontrolled plantar flexion following heel strike produces a classic, usually audible, "foot slap."

Orthotically, several options are commonly used to achieve shock absorption at the foot-ankle (Fig. 3–5). Metal uprights in an ankle-foot orthosis may contain a hinge joint

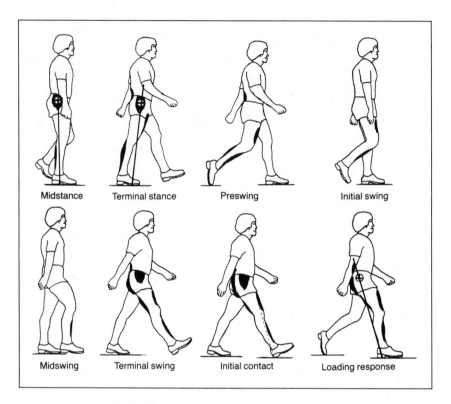

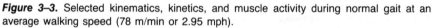

Figure 3–3. Selected kinematics, kinetics, and muscle activity during normal gait at an average walking speed (78 m/min or 2.95 mph).

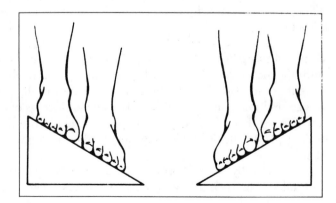

Figure 3–4. Surface adaptation of the foot-ankle.

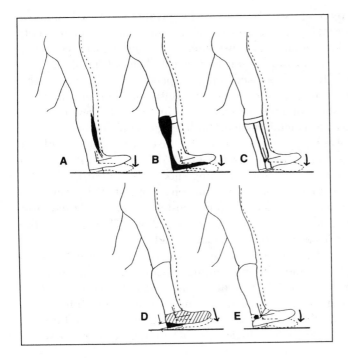

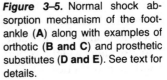

Figure 3–5. Normal shock absorption mechanism of the foot-ankle (**A**) along with examples of orthotic (**B and C**) and prosthetic substitutes (**D and E**). See text for details.

at which the motion into plantar flexion and "foot-flat" is controlled by a spring (Fig. 3–5C) that is incorporated into the joint. In a molded plastic ankle-foot orthosis (AFO), movement into plantar flexion is regulated by the posterior leaf spring portion of the orthosis (Fig. 3–5B).

Two possible prosthetic substitutes for foot-ankle shock absorption are depicted in Fig. 3–5; others will be described in later chapters. Figure 3–5D shows the widely used solid-ankle cushion-heel (SACH) prosthetic foot in which no motion occurs at the ankle but the shock absorption function is accomplished by compression of a foam wedge in the heel. Figure 3–5E depicts a "single axis" foot in which the amount and rate of plantar flexion following heel strike is regulated by the stiffness of a small rubber bumper or pad within the foot.

In general, since shock absorption is a mostly passive function in which the force of gravity is absorbed by body tissues, the elastic properties of metal, plastic, or foam can be used successfully to duplicate this function. It should be noted that reducing the speed of walking generally reduces the magnitude and rate of rise of the ground reaction force or "shock" imparted to the limb.

Effect on Center-of-Gravity Motion. The third function of the foot-ankle during ambulation is the effect that this segment has on movement of the body's center of gravity. In the sagittal plane, the center of gravity can be considered to be approximately one thigh length above the knee joint. Little can be done between the knee and the hip to smooth out the center of gravity path. Adjustments in limb length can be made, however, at the ankle. By progressively changing the pivot point of the foot-ankle from the apex of the heel to the ankle axis and then to the metatarsal area of the forefoot, the displacement path of the knee joint, and consequently the approximate center of gravity of the body, undergoes a smooth, minimal, vertical change (Fig. 3–6). One reason for, or at least a benefit from, decreased walking speed is that it reduces the vertical motions of the body's center of gravity and therefore the need for making large limb length adjustment using the foot-ankle. Figure 3–7 illustrates this point.

With an intact neuromusculoskeletal system, limb-length adjustments in early stance phase occur as a result of ankle plantarflexion, under the control of the dorsiflexor musculature, from heel strike until the foot is flat on the floor. The orthotic and prosthetic options that were discussed above regarding shock absorption usually also produce satisfactory limb-length adjustments during this phase of gait. Following foot-flat in an intact limb, gradually increasing activity in the posterior calf muscles controls and then completely limits the rotation of the tibia over the stationary foot, causing the rotation point to shift to the forefoot and the metatarsal heads.

Figure 3–8 illustrates several prosthetic and orthotic mechanisms used to limit continued rotation of the tibia over the foot, preventing a "drop-off" of the center of gravity in late stance. By definition a SACH foot has a solid ankle that allows no movement into dorsiflexion (Fig. 3–8B) so that beginning with midstance phase, the heel rises and weight is borne on the forefoot as the body continues to move forward. Another prosthetic option is shown in the single-axis foot in Figure 3–8C in which

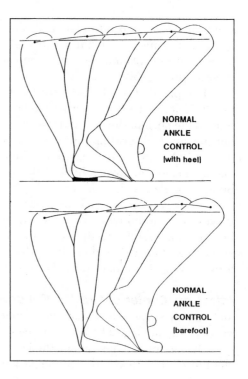

NORMAL ANKLE CONTROL (with heel)

NORMAL ANKLE CONTROL (barefoot)

Figure 3–6. Normal foot-ankle control and its effects on the movement of the knee path and therefore on the body's center of gravity.

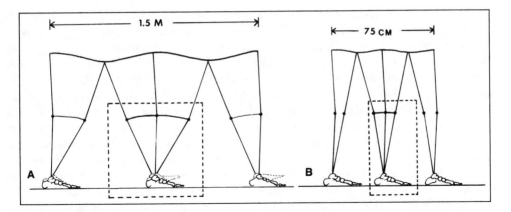

Figure 3–7. Knee path and approximate center-of-gravity path displacements during normal (**A**) and reduced (**B**) stride lengths associated with normal and reduced walking speeds.

resistance to motion is provided by an anterior rubber bumper whose compression limits the amount and rate of dorsiflexion motion. Orthotically the posterior leaf-spring action of a molded plastic AFO (Fig. 3–8D) and an anterior "stop" or spring used in the joint(s) of a metal upright orthosis (Fig. 3–8E) are examples of ways to externally control center-of-gravity movement in midstance and late stance.

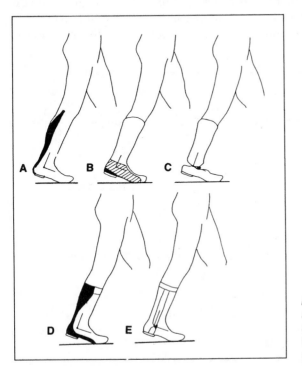

Figure 3–8. Normal mechanism (**A**) and examples of the use of prosthetic (**B and C**) and orthotic (**D and E**) devices to control the knee path and the center of gravity in late stance.

The normal progressive buildup in joint moments to eventually equal a steadily increasing external moment is a difficult function to produce artificially. In many instances motion into dorsiflexion in late stance is severely limited or is simply not allowed by the prosthetic or orthotic mechanism. This concept of a "fixed" or solid ankle raises the question about what ankle angle should be used to provide optimal gait performance for the user of the prosthesis or orthosis. From the point of view of the influence of the foot-ankle on the center-of-gravity movement, the angle at which the ankle is "fixed" has predictable effects. As illustrated in Figure 3–9, no resistance to dorsiflexion about the ankle joint results in a compasslike movement pattern of the knee-joint center and a severe drop-off of the center of gravity in late stance. Fixing the ankle in 10 or so degrees of plantarflexion causes the pivot point to shift to the forefoot relatively early in stance so that the center of gravity must "ride up" over the foot during late stance. A foot-ankle fixed in a neutral position has a similar but less dramatic effect than one set in plantarflexion, while an angle of slight dorsiflexion seems to produce a flatter trajectory but one with a slight drop-off.

Answering the question about which fixed ankle angle is ideal is not a simple matter. It requires consideration of at least two other foot-ankle functions, namely, knee stability and swing-phase shortening, to be discussed shortly. It is also important to remember that the slower walking speeds selected by many users of prosthetic and orthotic devices are accompanied by reduced requirements for limb-length adjustments at the foot-ankle.

Knee Stability. Support and movement of the mass of the body through space is in response to the ground reaction forces from the supporting surface. As the foot (or an assistive device) pushes against the ground, the reaction force against this push causes

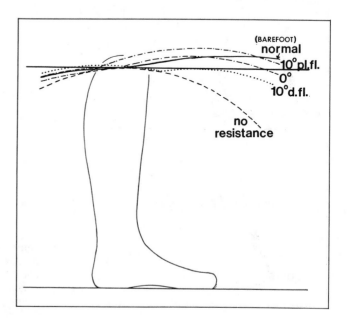

Figure 3–9. The effect of a "free" ankle and various "fixed" ankle angles on the knee path and the approximate center of gravity during stance.

the body to move (or remain stationary) in proportion to the magnitude and direction of the force. In the sagittal plane the "line of action" of the ground reaction force, on its path from the contact point under the foot to the body center of gravity, may pass anteriorly, posteriorly, or directly through the axis of the knee joint. If the ground reaction force passes through or anteriorly to the knee axis, the knee is considered to be mechanically "stable," since either no joint moment is required or the opposing moment is provided by passive posterior joint structures. If, however, the force line passes posteriorly to the joint axis, opposing moments must be provided by knee extensor musculature or else motion into flexion or knee "buckling" will occur. In this case the knee is considered to be mechanically "unstable." For example, walking in a crouched position with excessive knee flexion requires a great deal of knee extensor activity and is an exaggeration of a very unstable knee.

For individuals with compromised or absent knee function and reduced ability to control and/or maintain a flexed knee during weight bearing, configuration of an orthotic or prosthetic device to externally enhance knee stability may be very important. The factors that can affect the relationship of the supporting force line to the knee axis, and therefore its mechanical stability are the location of the body's center of gravity, the contact point (or center of pressure) under the foot, and the ankle angle. Figure 3–10 illustrates, during quiet standing, how knee moments can be affected by an AFO that "fixes" the ankle at a particular angle.[2] In the normal, unconstrained condition (Fig. 3–10A), the supporting ground reaction force line passes very close to the knee joint center so that minimal muscular control is required. Maintaining an attitude of dorsiflexion (Fig. 3–10B) shifts the knee-joint center forward and results in a knee-flexion moment that must be counteracted by appropriate activity in the knee extensor muscles. Maintaining a plantarflexed ankle angle (Fig. 3–10D) produces the opposite effect,

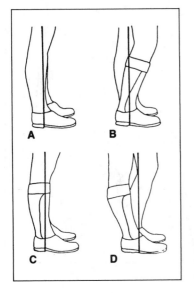

Figure 3–10. Examples of how knee moments can be affected by various "fixed" ankle angles in standing: (**A**) no orthosis; (**B**) dorsiflexed orthosis; (**C**) neutral orthosis; (**D**) plantarflexed orthosis.

shifting the knee center posteriorly behind the supporting force line so that the equal and opposite moment is provided by the posterior joint structures. The same principles apply to configuration of a prosthesis and are especially important in the case of an amputation above the knee where there is no attachment of the knee extensor muscles across the knee joint.

During gait, foot-ankle configuration becomes even more important to knee stability, since the ground reaction force is constantly changing in terms of both magnitude and direction throughout stance phase. By maintaining the foot-ankle in either plantar flexion or dorsiflexion it is possible to make the knee either more or less stable. Figure 3–11 illustrates these effects. The more extreme the angle in which the foot-ankle is maintained, the more dramatic the effect on knee stability. In patients who have difficulty maintaining the knee in extension during weight bearing, the prosthetic or orthotic foot-ankle can be fixed in a plantarflexion position so that the contact point tends to be anterior under the foot with the force line located near or anterior to the knee-joint center. Conversely, for patients with increased extensor tone or a tendency to severely hyperextend the knee, the foot-ankle can be maintained in dorsiflexion,

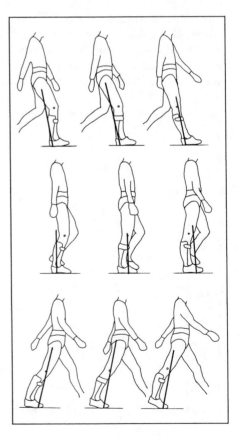

Figure 3–11. Examples of how knee moments can be affected by various "fixed" ankle angles during gait: (left column) ankle held in dorsiflexion by orthosis; (center column) ankle held in neutral position by orthosis; (right column) ankle held in plantarflexion.

tending to keep the contact point more posterior under the foot and the ground reaction force line closer to the knee joint center.

It must be remembered from the discussion in the previous section that fixing the ankle in a particular attitude also has consequences for the movement path of the body's center of gravity. A compromise must be reached to achieve adequate knee stability without excessively increasing the energy requirements associated with the center of gravity riding up or dropping off during late stance. The situation is further compounded by the need to control the foot-ankle during swing phase.

Swing-Phase Control. In normal gait the ankle is in a posture of approximately 20 degrees of plantar flexion when the toe leaves the supporting surface (Fig. 3–12). The ankle is returned to a neutral or near-neutral position by the time of midswing phase by contraction of the ankle dorsiflexors. Inability or failure to accomplish this motion results in an elongated limb requiring that other compensatory motions must occur elsewhere to prevent or to minimize dragging of the foot as it is brought forward.

Orthotically and prosthetically maintaining the foot-ankle in a near-neutral position often is not difficult, although there are exceptions. A near-neutral position usually provides adequate swing-phase control, but some compromises in selecting an optimal ankle angle often need to be made to also provide adequate knee stability and optimal center-of-gravity movement during stance.

Dragging of the foot or toe during swing phase does not necessarily indicate that a problem exists at the foot-ankle. As will be discussed shortly, adequate and coordinated

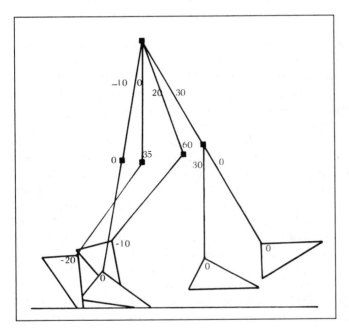

Figure 3–12. Motion occurring during a "normal" swing phase of gait.

motions of the knee and hip are also essential for clearance of the limb during swing phase.

Knee Functions During Gait

From a functional viewpoint three major functions of the knee during gait will be discussed: shock absorption, support, and limb shortening.

Shock Absorption. Concurrently with the shock absorption function of the ankle immediately following foot contact, the knee "normally" allows 15 or so degrees of controlled knee flexion to also absorb the "shock" of loading the limb. The quadriceps musculature eccentrically controls the rate of flexion and then concentrically returns the knee to nearly full extension by the time of midstance (Fig. 3–3). This slight knee motion also assists in smoothing the movement path of the center of gravity, which is at its lowest point during the double-support period and is changing direction from a downward motion to an upward motion at this time. Without this "yielding" of the knee, the limb is loaded more abruptly, causing a greater impact to the body tissues. Just as with most gait functions, reducing walking speed reduces the rate at which the limb is loaded and, consequently, the demand for controlled knee flexion in early stance.

Orthotically and prosthetically, shock absorption at the knee is difficult to provide with a mechanical device. Controlling the variable resistance needed to maintain a partially flexed, loaded knee, yet still provide adequate support and rapid swing-phase flexion, requires a sophisticated mechanism. Such components are likely to be complex, heavy, bulky, and expensive and are used only in a limited number of prosthetic applications.

Support. An important function provided by the knee during stance is support of body weight. As discussed earlier with regard to the influence of the ankle on knee stability, the line of action of the ground reaction force is of key importance. If that line is maintained anterior to the knee-joint axis, passive posterior structures provide the counteracting moment to prevent motion. If the force line is posterior, active knee extensors usually regulate the tendency for the knee to flex from body weight.

If active control of knee extension is compromised or absent, as is often the case in orthotic and prosthetic applications, the supporting force line must be maintained anterior to the knee to prevent knee buckling. A crucial time for establishing and maintaining knee stability is during early stance, when the ground reaction force tends to originate posteriorly under the foot and to pass posterior to the knee center. The relationship of the force line to the knee joint can be affected in three ways. The first method is to change the alignment of the device to affect the relationships among the origin of the force line under the foot, the knee axis, and the body's center of gravity. Changing the foot-ankle posture, as previously discussed, is one option (Fig. 3–11). Locating the knee axis more posteriorly and allowing hyperextension in a prosthetic system is another example (Fig. 3–13A). A second method for achieving greater knee stability is for the patient to locate the body's center of gravity more anteriorly by

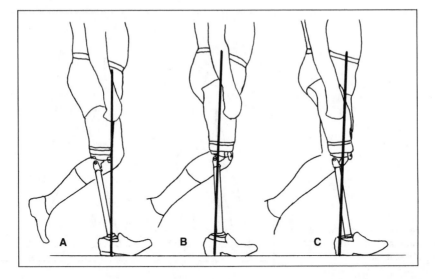

Figure 3–13. Techniques for achieving knee stability: (**A**) posterior location of knee axis and hyperextension of prosthetic knee; (**B**) move body's center of gravity forward by leaning, etc; (**C**) using hip extension moment to "dig in" with the heel and to tilt force line anteriorly.

leaning forward or using some other similar strategy to reconfigure the body segments (Fig. 3–13B). A third method is to produce an increased extension moment at the hip, causing the heel to "dig in" so that the force line tends to be angled more vertically than usual. Figure 3–13C illustrates this last technique.

The preswing phase is a period that may be particularly difficult with regard to support and knee stability for some users of prosthetic and orthotic devices. During this phase of "normal" gait, the knee joint begins to flex while still partially loaded (Fig. 3–14). As is discussed below, this preswing knee flexion is an important element in achieving a "normal" swing phase but may be very difficult or impossible for an individual with limited or absent control of the knee. Many times an individual with a prosthesis or orthosis will delay knee flexion in this phase of gait until the contralateral limb has been securely placed and loaded. Such delays result in a less smooth, usually slower, and less efficient gait pattern. Some sophisticated prosthetic knee units can successfully duplicate controlled yielding of the knee in preswing. In most prosthetic and orthotic applications, however, the point at which the knee begins to flex is determined by a combination of the three factors mentioned above: device alignment, center-of-gravity location, and hip moments.

Normally mediolateral control of joint moments at the knee is provided by the intrinsic structural integrity of the joint. When the knee joint has been affected by pathology or by trauma, structural deformities may result, and an external device may be needed to limit malalignment and pain and to improve function. Figure 3–15 shows an example of inadequate mediolateral support at the knee.

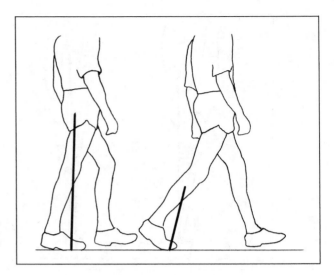

Figure 3–14. Normal terminal stance and preswing showing the partially loaded but flexed knee.

Limb Shortening. The most obvious function provided by the knee joint during normal gait is 60 to 65 degrees of flexion during swing phase to shorten the limb (Fig. 3–3). It should be noted that approximately one half of this motion occurs before the toe leaves the supporting surface (Fig. 3–14). If an individual, for whatever reason, does not get this start on knee flexion, it is virtually impossible to obtain the full knee flexion necessary for a normal swing. Consequently flexion during preswing is a necessary

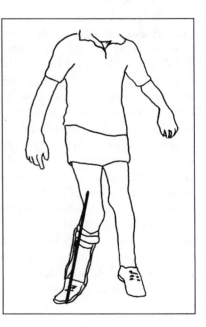

Figure 3–15. Example of inadequate mediolateral support at the knee.

precursor to adequate limb shortening during swing. Much of the power needed to flex the knee during swing comes from the hip flexor musculature and its effects on the compound pendulum configuration of the thigh and lower leg. By flexing the hip, the knee is secondarily also flexed. In some individuals and at faster walking speeds, the knee flexors may assist knee flexion in preswing. During preswing and initial swing, again depending on walking speed, the knee extensors normally contribute to limiting knee flexion and to initiating knee extension. In prosthetic and orthotic applications the challenge is to provide swing-phase control of the knee to replicate normal knee flexion and extension as closely as possible. Too much knee flexion in early swing results in excessive heel rise, while too rapid knee extension in late swing may result in a terminal swing impact as the knee reaches the limits of its motion. Clearly an external device that can accomplish normal control and adjust to various walking speeds is likely to be rather sophisticated. Some devices of this kind are available, especially for above-knee amputees. However, simpler devices, which are adjusted to a particular walking speed, are used in most cases.

Frequently, because of concerns for knee stability and patient safety, an orthotic or prosthetic device may use a locking mechanism that allows no motion at the knee. Sometimes, too, because of increased tone associated with neurologic deficits, some individuals maintain a rigid, fully extended knee during ambulation. The resulting "stiff-knee" gait poses some real problems during swing phase (Fig. 3–16). When preswing and swing phase knee flexion are absent, the individual is faced with the difficult task of advancing a relatively elongated limb during a relatively brief period. Temporal and distance asymmetries are very likely to result.

Since the vertical distance between the pelvis and the floor is less than the length of a stiff-knee limb, compensation of some kind must occur. Three common gait deviations often result from absent or inadequate knee flexion during the preswing and swing phases. They are entirely compensatory and may be present in different amounts and various combinations depending on the patient's status and abilities. Circumduction (Fig. 3–16B) involves using hip abduction during hip flexion to advance the limb in a semicircular path. This strategy increases energy requirements because of the added muscular power used for the additional lateral motion. Hip hiking (Fig. 3–16C) is a lateral tilting or relative abduction of the pelvis on the contralateral stance limb to provide a greater distance between the hip joint and the floor for the stiff limb to swing forward. This gait deviation is somewhat more energy consuming than circumduction, since it requires at least a slight vertical displacement of all the body segments except the contralateral stance limb. Vaulting (Fig. 3–16D) is the use of active plantar flexion during stance on the contralateral limb to elevate the entire body, thereby increasing the hip joint-to-floor distance for the swing limb. Vaulting is likely to be the most energy consuming of these three gait deviations. (A shoe buildup on one side can be used to prevent/simulate vaulting.)

Hip Functions During Gait

Hip functions during gait are somewhat simpler but are just as important as those of the foot-ankle and knee. In general, however, there are few prosthetic and orthotic devices that can adequately substitute for these functions.

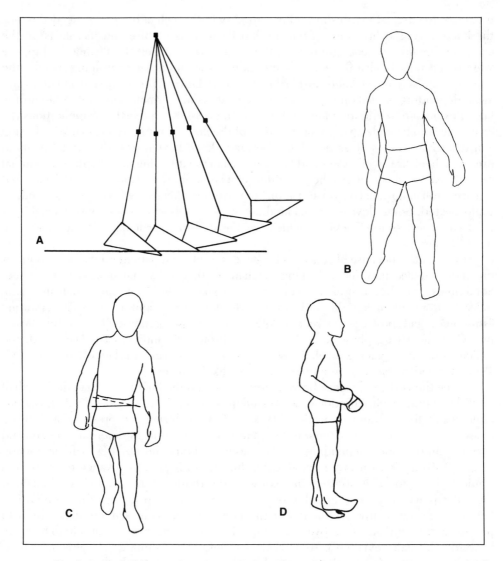

Figure 3–16. Stiff-knee swing phase: **(A)** the problem; **(B)** circumduction; **(C)** hip hiking; **(D)** vaulting.

Stance-Phase Extension. At the time of initial contact, the hip is normally in a position of approximately 30 degrees of flexion and progresses to a position of approximately 10 degrees of extension in terminal stance (Fig. 3–3). Since the ground-reaction force line tends to be anterior to the hip-joint axis in early stance, hip extensors are active to control the tendency of the trunk to rotate forward over the newly placed limb and to actively assist in hip extension. By midstance the force line tends to move behind the hip joint so that the hip flexors become active to control the amount and rate of hip extension and then to initiate the advance of the limb during swing.

Because hip extension during stance is principally an active, relatively powerful function, prosthetic and orthotic substitutes are difficult to devise and generally are not very successful, although there are exceptions to this statement. Compensatory gait deviations used by individuals with inadequate hip control may include backward leaning and lumbar lordosis (Fig. 3–17) in early stance (to keep the reaction force line closer to the hip joint center) and forward leaning and anterior pelvic tilting in late stance (to assist in the initiation of flexion during swing).

Swing-Phase Flexion. Beginning with preswing, the hip flexes to advance the limb through swing phase until initial contact and the next stance phase. As was mentioned previously, active flexion of the hip is required to attain adequate knee flexion. Additionally, the timing of hip flexion is important, since the hip must pass the neutral position before the knee begins extending, or clearance will be insufficient (Fig. 3–12). As with hip extension, swing-phase hip flexion is a difficult function to produce with an external artificial device. Individuals with hip flexion control problems often compensate with exaggerated motions of the pelvis and/or lower spine.

Mediolateral Stability. In the frontal plane the supporting force line is always medial to the hip joint throughout the stance phase of normal gait (Fig. 3–18A). Consequently the hip abductor group is active whenever body weight is borne on the limb, allowing

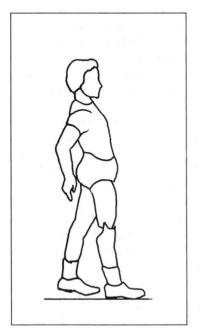

Figure 3–17. Lordosis as a compensatory gait deviation for inadequate control of the hip in early stance.

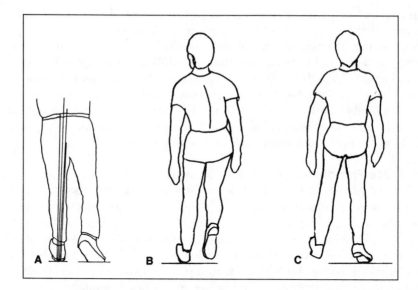

Figure 3–18. Frontal plane control of the hip: (**A**) normal showing medial floor reaction force vectors during stance; (**B**) lateral lean; and (**C**) abducted gait pattern as compensatory for inadequate control.

the pelvis to go through a slight (approximately five degrees) relative adduction on the femur. The hip abductors control the lateral shift of the center of gravity over the single limb, at first decelerating and then reversing lateral motion. In some applications, particularly with above-knee prostheses and hip-knee–ankle-foot orthoses, it is possible to provide mediolateral stability of the hip joint(s) with external devices.

Lateral leaning of the trunk toward the affected side is a common gait strategy for moving the force line closer to or through the joint so as to minimize the hip abductor requirements (Fig. 3–18B). The result is the classic Trendelenburg gait pattern. Another strategy adopted by some individuals is to use an abducted gait pattern to achieve a wider base of support (Fig. 3–18C). The advantage of such a pattern is that if control is lost, gravity will cause the body mass to move medially, a much safer situation than to get the body weight too far over the limb laterally and to fall away from the midline.

Other Causes of Gait Deviations

The preceding sections have discussed the principal functions accomplished by the lower limb during gait along with some common biomechanical causes of gait patterns that deviate from normal. There are certainly other reasons why a particular individual may choose to adopt a specific way of ambulating. Many of these will be presented in greater detail in Chapters 4 through 7. These reasons may include discomfort, feelings of insecurity, cosmesis, and a host of other physiologic, psychologic, and sociologic factors. It is the role of the health care provider to evaluate these factors as thoroughly as he or she can and to positively affect as many as possible.

REFERENCES

1. Stauffer S, Hoffer M, Nickel V. Ambulation in thoracic paraplegia. *J Bone Joint Surg.* 1978; **60**A(6):823–824.
2. Cook T, Cozzens B. The effects of heel height and ankle-foot orthosis alignment on weight line location: a demonstration of principles. *Orthot Prosthet.* 1976; **30**(4):43–46.

CHAPTER 4

Below-Knee Amputations and Prostheses

As mentioned in Chapter 1, lower limb amputations are 11 times more common than upper limb amputations. Leg amputations are divided into two general categories: below the knee and above the knee. Amputations below the knee joint are the most common level of lower limb amputation encountered today. This chapter will discuss different anatomic levels of below-knee amputation, the components commonly used in below-knee prostheses, how below-knee prostheses are suspended and aligned, and post-operative management of individuals who have experienced an amputation of the lower limb at the below-knee level. The chapter concludes with a consideration of energy expenditure and gait in below-knee amputees.

LEVELS OF BELOW-KNEE AMPUTATION

Below-knee amputations can occur within the foot, referred to as a partial-foot amputation; at the ankle, referred to as an ankle disarticulation, or Syme's amputation; or at any location through the tibia and fibula, usually simply referred to as a below-knee amputation.

Partial Foot Amputation

Various levels of partial-foot amputation are depicted in Figure 4–1. Amputations of the toes are a common form of partial-foot amputation. Toe amputations may be performed for a variety of reasons, including vascular disease, trauma, or secondary to a congenital deficiency. Except when the great toe is involved, little, if any, residual effect is usually noted, and the need for prosthetic restoration is small. Prosthetic restoration for cosmetic purposes is possible with the advent of modern plastics technology, although these prostheses are usually covered by a shoe.

An amputation at the transmetatarsal level creates a weight-bearing stump while minimizing the need for a prosthetic device. Transmetatarsal amputations are done for

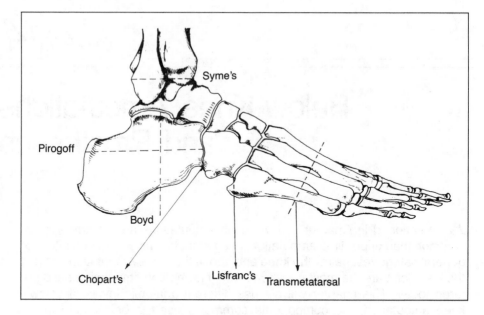

Figure 4–1. Partial foot amputation levels.

vascular as well as traumatic reasons. In either case a long, plantar flap, using the skin from the bottom of the foot, provides a good, weight-tolerant stump. Although the length of the foot lever is shortened following the amputation, it creates only a small functional impairment. Often the incorporation of a piece of spring steel in the sole of the shoe is sufficient to achieve good function. The gait of patients with a transmetatarsal amputation typically looks like they "fall off" at heel off due to the shortened anterior foot lever. Functionally this presents little difficulty, unless there is a need for forceful push off, as in walking quickly or uphill or in running.

The tarsal-metatarsal, or Lisfranc's amputation is named after the French surgeon Jacques Lisfranc and describes a disarticulation at the junction of the three cuneiforms and the cuboid. The anterior foot lever is further shortened compared to the trans-metatarsal amputation. Since the extensor mechanism is still intact, muscular balance about the ankle is maintained. The shorter the dorsum of the foot, the more difficult it becomes to keep a shoe on the remaining stump. The Lisfranc's level of amputation is the most proximal level that may be used without complications in young children. Studies have shown that the potential for ankle-flexion contracture increases when the amputation occurs above the insertion of the foot-extensor musculature, making functional use of a prosthetic device difficult.

Amputation at the midtarsal (Chopart's) level is named after the French surgeon Francois Chopart and leaves only the talus and calcaneus. Chopart amputation is not usually a level of choice, since the extensor mechanism will be absent and an unbalanced foot and deformity may occur.

Figure 4–2 shows an example of a partial foot prosthesis or shoe filler. The exact configuration will vary depending on the level of partial foot amputation.

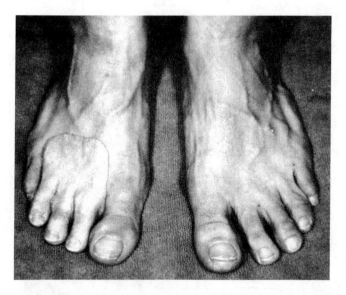

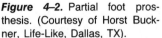

Figure 4–2. Partial foot pros-thesis. (Courtesy of Horst Buck-ner, Life-Like, Dallas, TX).

Ankle Disarticulation (Syme's Amputation)

The Syme's amputation is named for the famous Scottish surgeon James Syme, who practiced in Edinburgh between 1833 and 1869. Because he operated in the pre-Listerian and preanesthesia era, Syme needed a procedure that would allow him quick and sure amputation of the foot in cases of non-union fracture or life-threatening infection. Syme wrote that he could disarticulate the ankle in less than one minute and was successful in saving patients while retaining a stump that tolerates full weight bearing on the end (end bearing).

Syme's amputation is currently used for traumatic, congenital, and sometimes for vascular reasons. Wagner et al[1] reported up to 95% success rate using Doppler noninva-sive testing before two-stage Syme's amputations in dysvascular patients. Two-stage Syme's procedures disarticulate the foot in the first stage and close the wound, using the plantar skin, six weeks later. One of the indications for a Syme's amputation is that the patient must be a potential prosthesis user.

There are basically three types of Syme's prostheses: medial opening, designed by the Veterans Administration; posterior opening, designed by McLaurin in Canada; closed-panel or hidden-wall design, first described by LeBlanc[2] (Fig. 4–3). Hornby and Harris[3] in Toronto have questioned the long-term use of the Syme's level. In reviewing 68 patients with Syme's level amputations, he found that the majority of patients required proximal unloading of weight and distal relief from weight bearing. He concludes that a lacer-type socket is most efficient in relieving distal weight bearing.

The Syme's, or ankle, disarticulation level is also used in children secondary to trauma, congenital defects, or tumors. The Syme's offers a long, end-bearing stump, free from the problems of bony overgrowth often seen in pediatric amputations that transect long bones. The lower leg, particularly the fibula, tends to overgrow following transection. The fact that a patient may end bear and ambulate indoors without a prosthesis is often considered an advantage of the Syme's level. Davidson and Bohne[4]

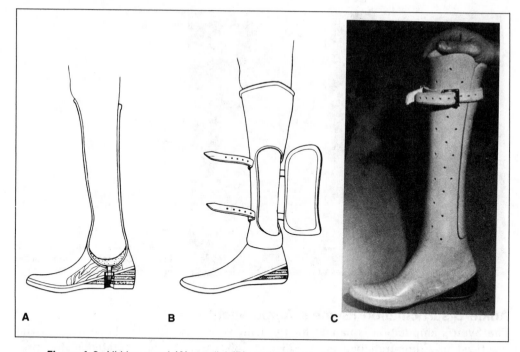

Figure 4–3. Hidden panel **(A)**, medial **(B)**, and posterior **(C)** opening Syme's prostheses.

reported positive results using the Syme's procedure in 23 children with a myriad of congenital problems. All patients walked within three months of operation, using standard Syme's prostheses. This group included patients with fibular dysplasia, proximal femoral focal deficiency (PFFD), and other problems. Leg-length discrepancies and foot/ankle deformities were the most common indications for Syme's amputation in children. Eilert and Jayakumar[5] compared the Boyd and Syme's level amputation outcomes in 34 children. The Boyd amputation transects the calcaneus longitudinally and fuses it to the distal tibia, thus preserving length. Although good results were found using both techniques, the best results occurred when the heel pad was plantigrade (neutral), occurring more often using the Boyd technique. All 34 patients were excellent prosthetic users, and all were fitted within three months of operation. Most could bear full weight on the end of the stump with or without the prosthesis.

In 1967 Sarmiento et al[6] reported on a new approach to the large, bulbous, uncosmetic Syme's amputation. Their modified approach, based on the premise that weight bearing can occur on the patellar ligament and on the medial flare of the tibia, eliminates the need for total end bearing in the prosthesis. By surgically shaving the malleoli, the overall stump circumference is reduced by one third without affecting the end-bearing qualities of the stump. The same posterior flap and heel pad is used to cover the stump and to close the wound. By making the end of the stump smaller, the need for a trap door in the prosthesis is eliminated. The resulting "hidden-panel" Syme's prosthesis looks smaller and is, therefore, more acceptable to many patients, particularly females.

Below Knee

Most authors and surgeons agree that the majority of lower limb amputations are largely related to severe vascular disease. The exact percentage is not known, but most agree that the percentage falls between 80% and 90%. Some authors suggest that the number of vascular-related lower-extremity amputations exceeds 33,000 per year in the United States. Since this is the case, most vascular amputations occur as elective procedures, that is, amputations performed by surgeons at an "elected" level, often at the below-knee level. Kay and Newman[7] reported that nationwide the below-knee amputation is more popular than the above-knee amputation. This fact represents a turnaround from the above-knee level, historically the more common procedure. This change may be related to two phenomena: the advent of noninvasive Doppler blood-flow detection equipment, and efforts by the American Academy of Orthopaedic Surgery following published studies demonstrating more successful rehabilitation when the amputation was done at the below-knee level. McCollough[8] states that 75% of patients with below-knee amputations related to vascular disease can become satisfactory users of a prosthesis, compared to less than 50% for the above-knee amputation. He cites the increased energy cost associated with the use of the above-knee prosthesis as the primary cause. He further states that many above-knee amputees prefer wheelchair locomotion, since it may be safer as well as less energy consuming. Moore et al[9] reviewed the literature and reported that between 48% and 77% of all below-knee amputations may be prosthetically rehabilitated. In his series of 18 cases, all healed primarily, and all were rehabilitated with a permanent prosthesis.

The below-knee amputation is a transmedullary amputation, resulting from a surgical ablation of the limb through the bone. This process creates the need for a prosthetic device designed to unload the weight proximal to the cut bone. Through-bone amputations do not tolerate weight bearing nearly as well as disarticulations, such as at the ankle or foot. Persson and Liedberg[10] investigated the ability of 69 amputees to tolerate end bearing. The average maximal weight bearing was 13 kg. Above-knee patients tolerated 13.7 kg, compared to 11 kg for the below-knee amputees. Vascular below-knee amputees averaged 10.7 kg. The ability of a stump to tolerate end bearing apparently does not change with time. Figure 4–4 illustrates different levels of below-knee amputation and the terms generally used to describe them.

Long Below-Knee Amputation. Most authors agree that saving all possible length is advantageous, often resulting in greater prosthetic function. Shea[11] reports that saving all possible length consistent with good circulation and wound healing is often difficult due to vascular compromise. Many authors prefer a midtibial length or longer and the use of the long posterior flap, or closure. This is thought to be a better approach than either an equal-length flap or a long anterior flap. Not placing the suture line on the very end of the residual limb makes prosthetic fitting easier.

Some authors report success using a side-to-side flap approach. Tracy[12] described a side-to-side, saggital flap approach. Persson,[13] in 1974, demonstrated the superiority of this procedure when compared to anterior and posterior flaps. Termansen[14] randomly compared this approach to the conventional long posterior flap described by Burgess et al.[15] Results indicated nearly equal rates of primary healing, although these rates were

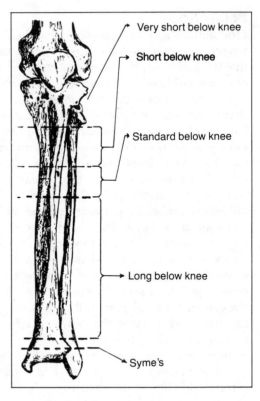

Very short below knee

Short below knee

Standard below knee

Long below knee

Syme's

Figure 4–4. Below-knee amputation levels. (From Northwestern University Prosthetic Orthotic Center, 1987, with permission.)

low when compared to other similar published works. There were no reported differences in outcome relative to limb fitting, occupation, or ambulation.

Medium Below-Knee Amputation. The length of a below-knee stump usually thought to be "medium" or standard in length is 5 to 6 in. This length was recommended by Burgess and Zettl[16] in 1969 for the elective below-knee amputation. A 3- to 5-in flap is left to cover the end of the stump. This skin flap, with continuous nerve and blood supply, is thought to assist the amputee with proprioceptive feedback and a sense of position of the stump within the socket. This standard-length stump allows for easy fitting of the patellar tendon-bearing (PTB) socket and any number of standard types of suspension, which will be discussed later in this chapter.

Short Below-Knee Amputation. The term "short" is usually used to describe a below-knee stump that is 4 cm or less in total length when measured from the medial joint line of the knee. Stumps of this length may present the prosthetist with great challenges. Considering the overall length and the small area of anterior skin upon which to unload the complete body weight, it is often necessary to use the distal end of the stump for weight bearing. As was mentioned earlier, end bearing, or loading the distal end of the stump, is not tolerated well and is usually not done. In the case of the very short below-knee stump, however, there is often no other choice. Flexion contractures may add to the difficulties encountered in the prosthetic fitting of the very short below-knee amputation. There is a greater risk of developing a flexion contracture when the stump is quite short, due in part to the imbalance created by the knee flexors and the tendency of patients with very short stumps to want to flex their knees while sitting or lying. Great care must be taken to prevent such a deformity from occurring.

COMPONENTS OF BELOW-KNEE PROSTHESES

The basic configuration in a below-knee prosthesis includes a socket, a spacer, and a foot. In addition, some form of suspension is necessary to keep the device in place on the residual limb. The spacer, between the socket and foot, may be made of either wood, plastic, foam, or a metal pylon, depending on the type of system used or the special needs of the patient. A "conventional" prosthesis is one that is often prescribed and fitted within a certain geographic area and often is specific to a given level of amputation. For example, a PTB socket with thigh corset and knee hinges might always be prescribed for below-knee amputees in spite of specific patient criteria or needs. A conventional fitting is usually not wrong, but often does not consider and include the patient's thoughts or needs in the prescription process. There is no universally accepted conventional prosthesis used equally in all areas of the country. Often the conventional prosthesis is dictated by the preferences or skills of the prosthetist in the area.

Prosthetic Feet

As presented in Chapter 3, the prosthetic foot should, ideally, substitute for the functions of the normal foot ankle. These functions include adaptation to uneven surfaces, shock absorption following heel strike, limb-length adjustments to smooth out the path of the body's center of gravity, stabilization of the knee, and limb shortening during swing. Clearly the prospect of substituting for all these functions with a simple, mechanical prosthetic foot is unrealistic. Several configurations present workable compromises and are commonly used in lower-limb prosthetics, both below-knee and above-knee.

The most commonly prescribed prosthetic foot used today in the United States is the solid ankle-cushion heel (SACH) foot (Fig. 4–5). The SACH foot has a wooden keel and a polyurethane foam heel wedge. The remainder of the foot is a poured polyurethane foam that will turn dark when exposed to direct ultraviolet light. For that reason many prosthetists will coat the foot with a plastic dip to prevent the foot from changing color. A survey of practice from 1973 to 1974 revealed that the SACH foot was used 81% of the time on below-knee amputations and 74% of the time on above-knee amputations.[17] A later study revealed that the SACH foot was used on 82% of all prostheses. Mechanically the SACH foot has no moving parts but simulates plantar flexion as the heel wedge compresses at heel strike and into early foot flat. Since there are no moving parts on the SACH foot, very little maintenance is required. However, occasionally a new heel wedge is needed if the heel becomes too soft. The prosthetist selects the heal-wedge density based on the weight of the patient. If the heel wedge is

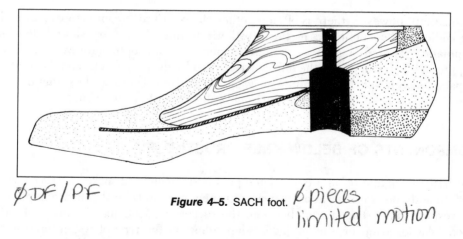

ɸDF/PF

Figure 4–5. SACH foot. *6 pieces*
limited motion

too stiff, foot flat is delayed, and knee instability may ensue. Conversely, in the case of weak knee extensors, a soft heel cushion or wedge is important to ensure that early and quick foot flat is achieved to maintain the floor reaction line in front of the knee axis, ensuring knee stability. Skinner et al[19] evaluated static load response of the heels of 30 standard SACH feet and found no difference between the "medium" and "regular" heel cushions. Consistency between feet of the same heel density rating was quite high. Skinner et al[19] concluded that all grades of heels of SACH feet were too stiff. SACH feet vary in weight from 445 to 490 g.

If one does not choose a SACH foot, a single-axis foot may be used. A single-axis foot allows limited motion in plantarflexion and dorsiflexion. It does so with the assistance of a plantarflexion bumper made of rubber or hard plastic. A single-axis foot may also contain an anterior dorsiflexion bumper, as shown in Figure 4–6. As the amputee places weight on the prosthetic foot at heel strike, the bumper allows plantarflexion of the foot, stopping it at the end of the allowable range. Generally the motion of the foot into plantarflexion is more rapid than with a SACH foot. Indications for the single-axis foot are thought to include an old prosthetic user who is accustomed to such a foot or the above-knee amputee who relies on the rapid plantarflexion of the foot to assist in knee stabilization. This concept will be further discussed in Chapter 5, which deals with above-knee amputations and prostheses. Doane and Holt[20] compared the differences between SACH and single-axis feet on eight male, unilateral, below-knee amputees. The results indicated that the single-axis foot permitted more plantarflexion and dorsiflexion than the SACH foot, but the time spent in each phase of gait was approximately equal.

In addition to the SACH and single-axis foot, a multiaxis foot is also commercially available. The multiaxis foot allows motion in dorsiflexion and plantarflexion as well as inversion and eversion. All motions are controlled by a system of bumpers similar to the bumpers previously described with the single-axis foot. The addition of inversion and eversion at the ankle allows for a small amount of movement of the foot for changes relative to the walking surface. Stability is afforded the amputee only at the extremes of motion in inversion and eversion, thus any movement in between those extremes is relatively uncontrolled. Otto Bock Orthopedic Industry, Inc. has added a torque rotator

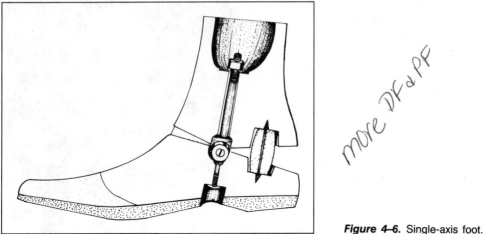

more DF & PF

Figure 4–6. Single-axis foot.

to the ankle components of the multiaxis foot, and the assembly is known as the Greisinger Manufacturer foot. The concept of torque rotation or conversion will be further discussed in Chapter 5 in the section dealing with above-knee prosthetic components.

Intuitively, amputees are thought to benefit from other than SACH feet, and much effort has gone into the research and development of multiaxis feet. However, very little clinical evidence exists to compare the benefits derived from a multiaxis foot with the increase in cost to the amputee. There is also increased weight at the end of the prosthesis as well as an increased need for maintenance, since multiaxis feet have a number of moving parts, which in time need maintenance or replacement.

Since about 1970 a number of new prosthetic feet have become available for use in below-knee prosthetics. These feet are not in large use today, as demonstrated by the component-use studies referenced previously, but are available to amputees and prosthetist to meet specific needs. One such change in prosthetic feet is the addition of sculptured toes to the available foot. Since many amputees prefer to wear sandals or open-toed shoes, the presence of the sculptured toes makes acceptance of the prosthetic foot easier. Additionally, the inclusion of the modular prosthesis concept into standard below-knee components has allowed the amputee to change feet to alter alignment. This allows shoes of different heel heights to be worn, making a great difference in the cosmetic acceptance and appearance of the amputee.

Studies by Burgess et al[21] of amputees running indicate that running requires some pronation and supination of the foot to allow the foot to bear weight on the lateral border following contact with the ground. To assist the amputee in this activity, the "Seattle foot" incorporates a leaf spring made of Delrin, which stores energy and aides in the push-off phase of running. The foot incorporates a rubber bumper angled at 22 degrees and an extension limitation cable that does not allow the foot to extend. Subjectively the foot allows more comfortable running and jumping. It weighs 595 g, or 1⅓ lb.

The latest entry into the prosthetic foot market is the "Flex-foot" (Fig. 4–7), which actually looks more like a ski than a foot. Developed by Van Phillips, the Flex-foot is

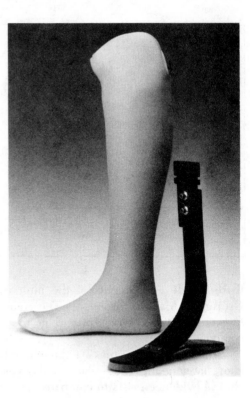

Figure 4–7. Flex-Foot. (From Flex-Foot, La-guna Hills, Calif with permission.)

made of a graphite laminate and has both heel and forefoot components. Early bio-mechanical studies by Wagner et al[1] suggest that using this foot provides a mechanical advantage to the amputee, even the geriatric amputee. Biomechanically, once the amputee has loaded the toe of the foot, the stored energy is returned at push off, thus assisting in propelling the amputee forward. Energy consumption studies by Nielsen[22] suggest that there is as much as a 20% energy savings by using the Flex-foot compared to a SACH foot, depending on the speed of the amputee's gait.

When comparing weights of some new feet, the Carbon Copy II is the lightest. Weighing only 415 g, it was purposely designed to go with the heavier Mauch hydraulic ankle. By comparison, the Seattle foot weighs 595 g, with Otto Bock's SACH foot weighing 445 g.

Whether the prosthetist uses the SACH, single-axis, multiaxis, or energy-storing foot in the components of the below-knee prosthesis, all foot/ankles are either glued and/or bolted to an ankle block in the prosthesis. In an exoskeletal system, the plastic laminate is added to the outside of the prosthesis to produce a cosmetically acceptable foot/ankle assembly. Endoskeletal systems, which have an aluminum or titanium pipe attached to the foot/ankle assembly, use a foam cover and stocking to provide cosmesis. This foam cover for the endoskeletal prosthetic system will be described in Chapter 5, which deals with above-knee prosthetic components, since a large number of endo-skeletal systems are fitted to amputees at the above-knee level.

The PTB Socket

Prior to the 1950s, most below-knee prostheses contained a plug socket, which consisted of a wooden, leather-lined ring, generally shaped in the form of a circle, into which the amputee placed the residual limb. Since the volume of a stump may change frequently, it was not uncommon for plug sockets to fit differently day to day or even hour to hour. The plug may be conceptualized as a cork in a bottle, and the distance that the cork is forced into the bottle depends on the size and shape of the cork as well as the force pushing the cork downward.

In contrast to the plug socket, the PTB socket, developed in the 1950s, uses total contact, a concept to be distinguished from end bearing. Total contact, in regard to the PTB socket, denotes a firm, but gentle force exerted by the socket over the entire area of the residual limb to contain the volume of the stump, not allowing distal portions to swell. Since many below-knee amputees have serious vascular diseases, it is essential that the prosthetist match the total-contact socket to the amputee's anatomy, to minimize distal edema problems. End bearing, on the other hand, connotes that the amputee is able to actually bear weight on the end of the residual limb. As was mentioned above, most through-bone amputations do not accept weight bearing without pain.[10]

The PTB socket is designed to have specific areas of weight bearing and specific areas of relief where very little or no weight is borne (see Fig. 4–8). Areas that are intended to accept weight are the patellar tendon (ligament), the medial flare of the anterior tibia, the lateral aspect of the residual limb, the pretibial muscle mass between the tibial crest and fibula, the lateral surface of the fibula distal to the head and proximal

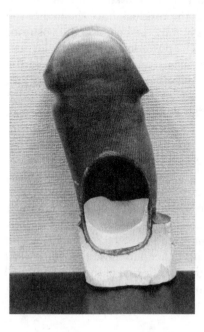

Figure 4–8. PTB socket, medial view, with exposure to demonstrate total contact on bottom.

to the cut end, and the popliteal fossa. The pressure-sensitive areas of the below-knee limb include the patella, tibial tubercle, crest of the tibia, anterodistal tibia, anterolateral tibial condyle, distal end of the tibia, fibular head, hamstring tendons, lateral distal fibula, common peroneal nerve, and saphenous nerve.

When the prosthetist prepares the positive model for the PTB socket, areas of weight bearing and relief are developed by modification to the model. If weight bearing is desired, plaster is removed from the positive model. Areas of relief receive extra plaster to develop recesses in the final socket. To assess the socket fit, a standing radiograph of the amputee in the socket may be used.

The PTB socket has essentially four sides or walls. Although the anterior wall is thought to be the primary weight-bearing wall, the other three walls play very important roles in the overall use of the PTB socket.

The top of the anterior wall is referred to as the anterior trim line. Generally the anterior trim line is finished in such a manner that the top bisects the patella. This bisection may be important as an anatomic landmark for evaluating proper socket fit. In some prosthetic designs the anterior trim line may exceed the proximal edge (or pole) of the patella as part of a supracondylar-suprapatellar suspension system, as will be discussed in a subsequent section. The medial and lateral walls are rounded in shape and rise above the proximal pole of the patella. These walls can be used to control the knee mediolaterally in stance phase.

The posterior wall functions to produce a counterpressure to maintain the anterior residual limb against the anterior wall for the purpose of weight bearing. Too great a distance between the front and back walls will not properly load the anterior wall. The height of the posterior wall depends on the overall length of the residual limb. The longer the limb, the lower the posterior wall can be to allow for full-knee flexion without the wall forcing the limb out of the socket. The shorter the residual limb, the higher the posterior wall to retain the soft tissue in the socket. Generally the height of the posterior wall is equal or just distal to the mid-patellar tendon. The posterior wall may be level or slanted downward from lateral to medial to clear the hamstring tendons. Usually the prosthetist attempts to enclose as much soft tissue as possible within the posterior wall so that these structures are not strangulated.

In addition to the features just described, the PTB socket is usually preflexed 8 to 10 degrees by the prosthetist as it is incorporated into the prosthetic limb. The purposes of preflexing the socket are to allow greater exposure of the anterior aspect of the residual limb for weight bearing; to maintain the knee joint in at least a neutral position, discouraging knee hyperextension; and to assist in the suspension of the prosthesis. Flexion of the socket is usually accompanied by slight dorsiflexion of the foot.

New amputees often need to be taught to walk in some knee flexion throughout the entire gait cycle, since it is not possible for an amputee with a preflexed socket to fully extend the knee. Therefore, a slightly shorter step may need to be taken, and a shorter initial contact period can be anticipated. It is important to keep in mind that since most below-knee prostheses incorporate a SACH foot, slight dorsiflexion of the solid foot will cause the knee to remain slightly flexed during stance, not allowing full extension or hyperextension. The greater the amount of flexion of the foot, the earlier in stance phase knee flexion will occur.

Special anatomic circumstances may dictate modifications to the typical prosthesis previously described. An amputee with a 35- or 40-degree flexion deformity of the knee can still be fitted with a functional prosthesis. However, the socket would need to be flexed to 40 or 45 degrees, making the leg very short and the step lengths even shorter.

PTB sockets may be of two basic types: hard sockets or sockets made with liners. Liners provide an interface between the stump sock and the socket and are preferred by some prosthetists and many amputees. They are thought to provide somewhat of a cushion, thus offering the amputee a more comfortable fitting. Indications for the use of a socket liner are often a very bony residual limb and one where weight bearing may place undue force on the tibia, usually on the crest. In children, liners are often used to offer greater flexibility of socket fitting as the child grows. As growth occurs, stump socks are removed. When no more socks can be removed, the liner is removed, making the socket larger and allowing the amputee more time between socket fabrications. Socket liners may be fabricated from many different materials ranging from leather to plastic. Current materials used for socket liners include Pelite, Spenco, Plastazote, and leather. Koepke et al,[23] in 1970, described a silicone gel socket covered with horsehide. This gel socket was indicated for amputees with skin problems such as skin grafts, extensive scars, and limbs without sensation. This silicone gel insert, developed at the University of Michigan, distributes pressure evenly and is thought to lessen shear forces that can contribute to skin breakdown and ulceration. Usually when a socket liner is worn the amputee first dons the liner and then inserts the liner into the socket.

In the PTB hard socket, stump socks are nearly always used as an interface between socket and skin. They may be wool or synthetic and serve to add volume within the socket as limb volume decreases. The smaller the limb the more plies of sock necessary. Socks come in many sizes and thicknesses, ranging from 1 to 6 ply.

The Prosthetic Skin

The external covering, or prosthetic skin, of the prosthesis may be either plastic laminate or a heavy cotton stocking over foam, depending on the type of prosthesis. The function of the prosthetic skin is to cover the device in a cosmetically acceptable manner. With an exoskeletal type, a combination of fiberglass stockinet and thermal-setting plastic combine to provide the amputee with a hard plastic shell, similar to the shell of a turtle. This prosthetic skin provides the structural stability for the prosthesis as well as protection for the stump and component parts. With an endoskeletal system the actual structure of the device is afforded by an aluminum or titanium pipe and connectors, with the cosmetic restoration produced by a foam cover and a heavy cotton sock. The polyurethane foam cover is shaped by the prosthetist based on circumferential measurements of the amputee's remaining limb. It should be understood that the exoskeletal type of hard plastic shell is far more durable and acceptable to amputees who work outside or to amputees who work in situations where the cosmetic cover and sock would be exposed to grease, dirt, or any activity that could cut the sock and foam cover.

Preparatory Prostheses

A preparatory prosthesis is any prosthesis that is not permanent or "definitive" and allows ample opportunity for modifications. The purpose of any preparatory prosthesis is to allow early ambulation at an efficient and safe level and yet allow for the rapid changes in volume that often occur in the days and weeks postoperatively. Preparatory prostheses may be made of many materials, including plaster, wood, plastic, and metal. Preparatory prostheses often do not cost as much as a finished limb but allow the patient to walk safely in a custom-fabricated socket (Fig. 4–9). Preparatory prostheses will be discussed further in the section on rigid dressings.

When using modular prosthetic component systems, the endoskeletal tube may also serve as the temporary prosthesis. This allows the care team to begin training with the prosthetic device and to withhold final cosmetic restoration pending the results of the training. In this case the "temporary" is also the permanent limb, with the difference being the completion of the cosmetic cover.

SUSPENSION OF THE BELOW-KNEE PROSTHESIS

Suspension refers to the components and design features used to hold a prosthesis in place while the amputee ambulates and performs other functional activities. Suspension of the below-knee prosthesis may take many forms. It is desirable to use the easiest and simplest possible form of suspension, since most amputees resist the addition of straps, belts, and the like, particularly if they are functionally unnecessary. The anatomy of the knee and thigh often determine the ease with which the prosthesis may be suspended.

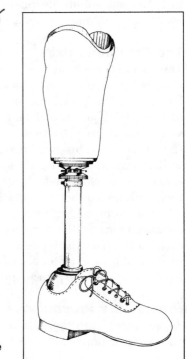

Figure 4–9. Below-knee preparatory prosthesis, with removable pylon and SACH foot.

Normal anatomy of the thigh allows many suspension applications that center around the fact that the femoral condyles provide a useful attachment location. Amputees who are overweight or have excessive soft tissue around the thigh and knee, make the suspension of below prostheses more difficult. Figure 4–10 shows examples of different types of suspension, as discussed in the following sections.

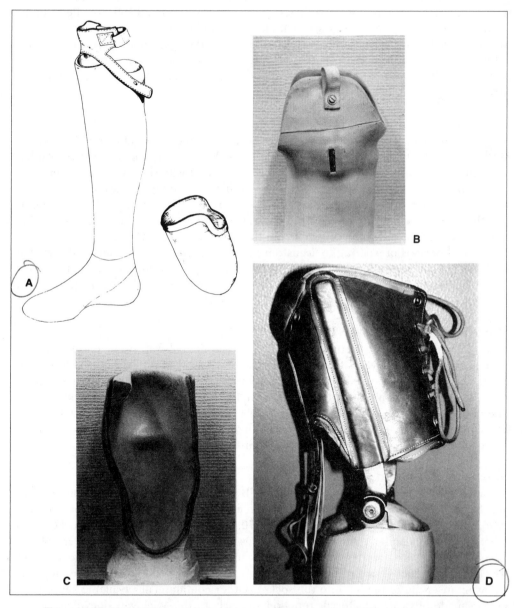

Figure 4–10. Various forms of below-knee prosthetic suspension. (**A**) supracondylar cuff; (**B**) removable medial wall or brim; (**C**) removable medial wedge; (**D**) thigh corset with knee joints.

The Supracondylar Strap

One of the most frequently used means of suspension in the below-knee prosthesis is the supracondylar strap (Fig. 4–10). The supracondylar strap is usually made of leather, vinyl, or other plastic and is riveted to the medial and lateral walls of the socket and placed around the popliteal area. The supracondylar strap classically either buckles or closes using Velcro, so that only one hand is required to fasten it. In some cases the supracondylar strap may not be sufficient to completely suspend the prosthesis in all circumstances, and an auxiliary waist belt may be added to ensure adequate suspension. An additional feature of the supracondylar strap is that it may act to limit hyperextension of the knee during stance phase. A disadvantage to the supracondylar strap is that it may present a high amount of force in the popliteal space, particularly while the amputee is sitting or when the knee is flexed to 90 degrees.

The Medial Wedge

Another means of suspending the PTB prosthesis is the removable medial wedge. Medial wedging technique involves a soft, pliable, often leather or plastic wedge inserted by the amputee inside the medial wall of the prosthesis in the crevice created by atrophy of the vastus medialis. Once the residual limb and wedge are in place in the socket, no further straps are necessary. The lateral wall must be rigid and unyielding so that the medial-wedge pressure pushes the residual limb against the lateral wall. This compression may cause some discomfort in the early wearing periods, often necessitating gradual periods of wearing to accustom the medial aspects of the leg to the wedge and its pressure. Sometimes the medial wedge is incorporated into the medial side of a socket liner so that no other removable wedge is necessary, providing the amputee with a very cosmetic PTB prosthesis that is self suspending.

The Removable Medial Wall

When the medial wedge used for suspension is the medial wall itself, one has a PTB suspension variant known as the removable medial wall (RMW), or removable medial brim. This type of suspension allows the amputee to remove the entire medial wall, to insert the leg, and then to insert the medial wall into a steel channel laminated into the side of the prosthesis. The removable wall has a wedge-shaped protrusion formed on it that conforms to the medial musculature of the knee. Through both swing and stance phase, the wedge in the medial wall maintains the limb in place.

Sleeve Suspension

A relatively new form of suspension for the PTB prosthesis is sleeve suspension. Sleeves may be made of many different materials such as rubber, knitted cotton or elastic, or a cotton-polyester blend. Koepke et al,[23] in 1970, described the silicone gel socket used for problematic residual limbs, or difficulties in pressure distribution. Part of the "Michigan leg" was a rubber sleeve that was used for suspension. The rubber sleeve attaches to the socket of the prosthesis and is pulled over the knee by the amputee following insertion of the leg into the socket. Other commercially available suspension sleeves made of various materials function similarly to the Michigan sleeve. Although the rubber sleeve may not be used in all climates, it is a viable form of suspension when heat and humidity are not a problem. These sleeves are not useful when the amputee will be walking over muddy ground or when the possibility of excessive downward forces on the prostheses exists.

Thigh Corset and Knee Hinges

Another form of suspension for the below-knee prosthesis is the thigh corset and knee hinge. This form of suspension is quite bulky and is used only when necessary. Usually the amputee using this form of suspension has some instability of the knee and uses the knee hinges as an orthosis (see Chapter 7). The instability may be either mediolateral or anteroposterior. Other candidates for thigh corset and knee-hinge suspension are amputees whose skin on the residual limb is unable to tolerate the applied forces and who need an additional area over which to distribute the forces. This situation occurs in amputees doing heavy lifting, in juvenile diabetics, in patients with systemic lupus erythematosis (SLE), and in rheumatoid arthritics. Knee hinges used with PTB sockets may be either single axis or polycentric. Polycentric hinges have a moving center of rotation and are thought to act more like the normal anatomy of the knee joint. For this reason polycentric hinges are preferred by many amputees, since undue pressure from socket binding can be avoided.

MANAGEMENT OF THE RESIDUAL LIMB

An important part of postsurgical care of the amputee is devoted to managing the residual limb or stump. This management consists of simultaneously attending to wound healing and to shaping and conditioning the stump for its new function of weight bearing. Two techniques have developed as important aspects of residual limb management: application of a rigid postsurgical dressing and compression wrapping.

Rigid Dressings

The concept of early prosthetic fitting dates back to the early 18th century and probably long before. During World War I and II, early temporary prostheses were made from plaster and broom handles. These prostheses were used successfully throughout Europe. In the 1950s, interest in the United States in active mobilization of the residual limb and the development of the elastic bandage sparked a renewed interest in early prosthetic fitting. In 1957 surgeons first used plaster and pylons to serve as provisional or temporary prostheses. Early experience with this system confirmed what had been written years before—that walking on an immature stump had positive effects on stump maturation. In 1958 the first-recorded, immediate, postoperative prosthetic fitting occurred while the patient was on the operating table.[24] The technique was soon refined and popularized in this country by Burgess.[16]

The components of the rigid dressing as described by Burgess[16] include (1) Lycra Spandex stump sock, (2) Scived relief pads for tibia and patella, (3) elastic plaster, (4) regular plaster, (5) waist belt and suspension strap, and (6) pylon and SACH foot assembly. The stump sock is pulled over the wound, covering the distal stump with sterile lamb's wool to allow for wound drainage. Beveled felt pads are placed on the patella and on both medial and lateral sides of the crest of the tibia. Elastic plaster is wrapped over the stump followed by regular plaster. A suspension strap is encased in the plaster near the end of the procedure, and a waist belt is placed on the patient. The patella covering is removed, and any extra plaster is cut away. Drying time is 12 to 24 hours, depending on temperature and humidity. The pylon and SACH foot are added, and the final pylon adjustment is done with the patient standing.

The results attributed to the use of the rigid dressing in the middle to late 1960s were better wound healing, need for fewer postoperative narcotics, earlier ambulation, less edema, and the psychological advantage of never being without a limb. Through the 1960s and early 1970s there were many reports concerning the use of new surgical techniques that benefitted the dysvascular amputee. Few, if any, studies were sufficiently controlled to allow fair evaluation of the influence of any one aspect of new treatment procedures. Many of these new procedures improved patient care simply by emphasizing the saving of the knee joint, particularly in the elderly. In was not until Mooney[25] published his work in 1971 that the use of immediate postoperative rigid dressings in the dysvascular amputee was questioned. In 182 cases of below-knee amputation on dysvascular patients, he concluded that rigid dressing and ambulation were good and probably contributed to the overall well-being of the patients. However, he also concluded that ambulation within the first two to four weeks may deter wound healing. In 1977, Baker et al,[26] in a prospective study, reported evidence that the use of the rigid dressing procedure did not result in a higher percentage of wound healing in vascular diseased patients with below-knee amputations. Wound healing was reported as 85% using the rigid dressing and 83% using soft dressings. However, patients with rigid dressing were discharged on postoperative day 7.3 on the average, whereas patients with soft dressings were discharged in an average of 14.7 days. Patients with rigid dressings began ambulation using a prosthesis at postoperative day 29.6, whereas patients with soft dressings began at postoperative day 35.5.

Rigid dressings with pylons are intended to be used for partial weight bearing. Slight dorsiflexion of the prosthetic foot usually allows the patient to have a smoother advance through stance phase during early ambulation. The pylon is often shortened an inch or so to allow for swing phase without circumduction, vaulting, or hip hiking. The pylon/foot assembly may be removed while the patient is in bed. This avoids the tendency for the hip to passively externally rotate secondary to the round heel of the foot. The combination of a rigid dressing and pylon is one form of a temporary prosthesis. Generally, temporary prostheses are used in cases where large volume reductions in the stump are anticipated. As long as the distal stump has a larger circumferential measurement than the proximal measurement, a plaster dressing may well be the treatment of choice.

Currently, rigid dressings with or without pylon are generally in use throughout the United States, and the technique may be learned by anyone. The rigid dressing is generally applied by a prosthetist or surgeon, although in some facilities it is applied by a physical therapist or orthopaedic physician assistant.

Compression Wrapping

Compression wrapping is a procedure that aids in the shrinking and maturation of the residual limb or stump. It is often performed using rubber or synthetic elastic wraps and is usually taught to the patient or significant other so that it may be carried out in the patient's home. Compression wrapping is part of a system often referred to as a soft dressing. Soft dressings usually consist of cotton-mesh gauze wrapped over the stump, followed by a compression wrapping often referred to as an "Ace" wrap. Compression wraps are commercially available in many sizes and in a number of different materials. Generally wraps are 2, 3, 4, and 6 in wide. The length may vary, and it is often necessary to sew two wraps together to produce one longer wrap. Generally, compression wraps are applied to create pressure gradients, with more pressure being applied distally and less pressure being applied as the wrap proceeds proximally. Wrapping continues indefinitely, as the maturation process frequently takes 9 to 12 months, and often longer.

There are two basic techniques of application for the compression wrap. One is called the recurrent and the other a figure-of-eight. The recurrent wrap is started front to back and is then held while the wrap is started in a figure-of-eight motion. This technique is often difficult for patients to master. Instead, it may be easier to teach the figure-of-eight style, since it requires only two hands and is very simple to learn (Fig. 4–11). Whichever technique the amputee uses, pressure should be applied on the oblique turns and not on the circular turns. The result of applying too much pressure on the circular turns is a tourniquet, which may compromise the viability of the stump as well

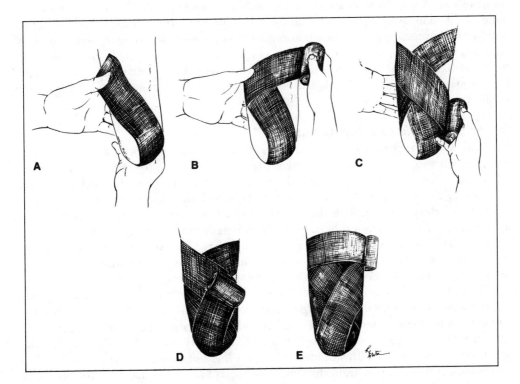

Figure 4–11. Stump wrapping for below-knee amputation using modified figure-of-eight technique.

as delay prosthetic fitting due to large amounts of "boggy" edema. The wrap should extend above the knee and above the proximal pole of the patella. This allows for a consistent shrinking of the entire stump as well as affording some degree of suspension for the wrap. Wrinkles in the wrap can cause skin problems, and care should be taken to avoid them. Patients should be discouraged from active knee-flexion exercise while the wrap is in place. This will serve to increase the pressure over the patella and tibial tubercle and will also lead to an ultimate loss of suspension of the wrap. Isherwood et al[27] studied the pressure associated with the use of soft dressings and, particularly, elastic compression dressings. Results of their work indicate that the greatest pressure on the below-knee residual limb occurs over the tibial tubercle. In fact, the mean pressure for both skilled and unskilled bandagers was greater by 28 mm Hg over the tibial tubercle, ranging from 39 to 67 mm Hg.

An alternative to a rolled compression wrap is a shrinker sock, which is typically an elastic sleeve with one end tapered and sewn shut. The sock is pulled over the residual limb and is held in place using tape or Velcro. Shrinker socks are available in many sizes, thicknesses, lengths, and knittings. The advantages cited for using the shrinker socks compared to compression wraps are ease of application and no need for understanding or learning wrapping techniques. The cost of the device is more than most compression wraps but may be worth the investment when dealing with homebound patients who have difficulties with stump wrapping. Varghese[28] reported comparisons of compression wraps, shrinker socks, and a modified shrinker sock. The modification was done based on measured pressure readings taken from the stump. Results indicated that patients had excessive pressures when regular compression wraps were used. The best results came from the modified shrinker sock, which showed increased venous return in the residual limb. The sock maintained pressure longer and was easier to apply. Single-knit shrinker socks delivered less-than-ideal pressure and deteriorated following several washings.

Other Stump Maturation Options

Wu and Krick[29] reported on an alternative to either conventional rigid dressings or compression wraps. The removable rigid dressing (RRD) involves the use of a plaster shell, socks, a stockinet sleeve, and a thermoplastic supracondylar cuff. Tube socks are used under the plaster shell to accommodate volume loss. Additionally the cast may be safely used while standing with the assistance of a simple car jack. The RRD is usually applied following the removal of the first thigh-length rigid dressing. It may, however, be used with both recent and long-term amputees. The removable rigid dressing reportedly saves 90 days of hospital stay by eliminating many breakdowns of the skin often seen in below-knee amputees using compression wraps.

In addition to the postoperative dressings or systems previously discussed, other options exist. These options may be generally referred to as soft, or semirigid. Although soft dressings of gauze and cotton are commonly used with a more delayed prosthetic fitting, 80% healing success was reported by Gay and Heard[30] when the soft dressing was used in conjunction with surgical techniques that left a long posterior skin flap. The two principal types of semirigid dressings are the Unna's paste boot and the air splint. Unna's paste boot is a zinc oxide-impregnated gauze that is commercially available like plaster. The boot never hardens but provides some external pressure to the stump while giving it some shape. The procedure for application has been described by Ghiulamila.[31] Felt relief pads are used along the crest of the tibia in a way similar to a plaster rigid dressing. Unna's paste boot does not allow for any swelling and may be applied by anyone knowledgeable in the technique.

Writing primarily in British publications, Little[32] reported on the postoperative use of an air splint. Use of the air splint is said to facilitate early ambulation and balance training and to allow partial weight bearing on the recently amputated limb. Little's[32] article, published in 1970, described the use of air splints on five patients, all dysvascular and all having long posterior flaps. Following closure of the wound, the air splint was applied and inflated to a pressure of 25 mm Hg. Sweating under the splint was noted as a nuisance, and the addition of a walking pylon was reported to be difficult, if not impossible. Little does not claim that the air splint system is better or even equal to the rigid dressing system. He does, however, believe it to be easier to apply and use. In the United States, use of the air splint was reported by Kerstein[33] and Sher.[34] Both cite the same advantages as Little, plus the ability to see the wound and to inspect it at any time without the problems of removing and reapplying a plaster cast. The technique of Kerstein involves a stump sock and felt relief pads, similar to a plaster rigid dressing. Kerstein reported results on 11 patients indicating, as did Little, that no pylon attachment was possible with the air splint. Sher first used the air splint when no prosthetist or early prosthetic program was available.

Other Factors Affecting the Residual Limb

It is not possible to describe in detail all the possible stump conditions that might be encountered in an active prosthetics/orthotics clinic. However, this section will discuss some general considerations that may affect the course of treatment or the indications for specific components or modifications.

The presence of a break in the skin or a sore does not, in and of itself, contraindicate the use of a prosthesis while the sore is open or even draining. While physician preference may dictate some situations, it is imperative to understand why the sore or ulcer first appeared. Appropriate steps may then be taken to relieve the area, and the patient may return to limited ambulation, always being careful not to increase the size or severity of the sore. This approach may be difficult for some patients and families to grasp, since many equate skin sores with potential trouble and with the series of events that may have led to the amputation in the first place.

Burns, either thermal or electrical, can result in limb amputations and often leave scars that can be difficult to manage. If the scarring occurs on the lower extremity, the need to bear weight on that extremity may make the prosthetic fitting fraught with skin breakdown, particularly in the early weeks and months following the amputation. As the skin contracts, the chance of ulceration increases. Careful and watchful follow-up and well-educated family members are very important.

Perhaps the most common problem dealt with in the follow-up of patients with amputations is edema. No other problem is seen so frequently and is such a source of frustration for amputees and their families. Since the great majority of amputations are done for vascular reasons, it should not be surprising that the postoperative problem list includes edema. As was mentioned in the section describing the PTB socket, edema can affect socket fit and lead to ulceration when bony prominences are not resting in their designated places within the socket. It also can confuse the amputee regarding the correct number of plies of stump socks to wear.

In cases of severe diabetes or other vascular conditions as well as any of a group of peripheral neuropathies, normal feeling in the stump is diminished or lost altogether. When this occurs, skin breakdown is often persistent. Important factors involved in evaluating these situations are the type and fit of the socket, the adherence to recommended amounts of ambulation, and the use of proper numbers of plies of stump socks. In some instances nothing can prevent ulceration, and patient management is from one episode to another. In other situations more proximal unloading of weight is helpful. This may take the form of a thigh lacer, which is reported to relieve as much as 40% of the patient's weight from the PTB socket. In extreme cases patients are placed in a quadrilateral socket, similar to the sockets used with above-knee amputations, as described in the next chapter. Additionally, special liners used inside the socket can help to distribute the weight more evenly. Adequate length of the residual limb can be important in the prevention of ulceration by affording a large surface area for weight bearing, resulting in less force per unit area.

In those cases where a marked flexion contracture exists and conservative measures fail to improve the clinical picture, a bent-knee prosthesis may be fitted. Such a device usually incorporates thigh corset and knee-hinge suspension and allows the patient to walk with the knee in a bent or flexed position, taking all the weight on the anterior tibial aspects of the stump. A cosmetic problem exists when the bent-knee prosthesis is used. However, in those few cases where no other device will function, this option should be considered. Clinical experience dictates that the patient should be fully informed beforehand as to exactly what the device will look like.

ALIGNMENT OF THE BELOW-KNEE PROSTHESIS

The term alignment refers to the physical relationship between the socket and the prosthetic foot. Much attention is paid to alignment to attain the optimal function for the amputee, particularly during stance phase with the amputee in a position of full weight bearing. Proper alignment will provide the amputee with the opportunity to comfortably bear all weight on the limb without undue forces causing either pain or ulceration.

Static Alignment of the Below-Knee Prosthesis

As discussed in Chapter 2, alignment occurs in two phases: static, or bench, and dynamic. Static, or bench, alignment is the configuration in which the prosthetist places the prosthesis before the initial limb fitting. This usually occurs in the office of the prosthetist and before any visit to the physician or physical therapist. The bench alignment will usually allow most amputees to begin ambulation. Since bench alignment is almost always done using an adjustable (temporary) leg, changes may be made while the amputee walks to provide the most comfortable and efficient gait possible.

One of the primary devices used by the prosthetist in bench aligning a prosthesis is a plumb bob, a pointed weight on the end of a string that provides a true vertical reference. The prosthetist aligns the prosthesis so that a plumb line hung from the center of the posterior wall will fall about one-half inch lateral to the center of the heel of the shoe of the prosthesis, as seen in Figure 4–12. Thus the foot will be one-half inch inset from true vertical. This insetting of the foot in bench alignment accommodates for the bowing of the tibia, helps load pressure-tolerant areas, and allows for a reasonable distance between the heels during gait. As was discussed in Chapter 3, the narrower the base of support the less energy consuming the gait.

In the anteroposterior plane, the prosthesis is aligned so that a plumb line from the center of the lateral wall will fall just anterior to the frontmost edge of the heel, a location sometimes referred to in prosthetics as the breast of the heel. Although there is no ankle in a SACH foot, the plumb line would pass just anterior to it if there were one.

Dynamic Alignment of the Below-Knee Prosthesis

Following acceptable bench alignment, dynamic alignment occurs while the amputee is walking and in full weight bearing on the involved side. The guiding principle in dynamic alignment is that the pylon or pipe of the alignment device is perpendicular to the floor when the amputee is in full weight bearing. This determination must be made both from the front and back as well as from the side. Using the adjustable jig, the prosthetist or therapist adjusts the alignment, attempting to optimize the amputee's gait pattern. Experience is necessary to perform this alignment and can be learned with the supervision and assistance of an experienced prosthetist. It is important to remember that any changes made with the adjustable leg are likely to alter the forces on the limb, so a thorough understanding of the process should precede any attempted changes in alignment. Many prosthetists prefer that all changes in alignment be made in their office. However, a more ideal working relationship among health care professionals

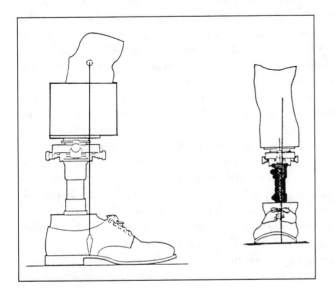

Figure 4–12. Bench alignment for a PTB prosthesis.

allows adjustments to be made by a knowledgeable therapist throughout the amputee's initial gait-training period. This arrangement is more efficient for the amputee and saves much time and effort for the physical therapist.

FUNCTIONAL TRAINING OF THE BELOW-KNEE AMPUTEE

Individuals who undergo amputation for vascular insufficiency are generally deconditioned, diabetic, and have been hospitalized or at home for a long time trying to heal a long-standing foot or lower-leg ulcer. Silbert[35] reported that 41% of the diabetic amputees he studied lived longer than three years postoperatively but that 51% of those surviving the surgery lost their remaining limb within five years. Mazet[36] reported similar results, stating that a second amputation occured 33% of the time within five years of the first. Whitehouse et al[37] stated that the dysvascular amputee is more likely to die than to lose the remaining limb. McCollough et al[38] reported that in 27 cases of bilateral below-knee amputations, 20 lost the second limb within two years and seven before six years. In view of this data, amputees should have well-fitting, protective, and sometimes custom-made insoles or entire shoes to make every effort to preserve the contralateral extremity. A double-depth, large, toebox shoe is helpful in this regard. By removing the double-depth inlay, material such as Plastazote is easily placed in the shoe to aid in pressure distribution.

Preprosthetic Care

The postoperative care following amputation surgery is a team effort by all parties concerned. It is important for the patient's success that the care be consistent with what was promised preoperatively and that all parties continue to communicate. In large general hospitals it is convenient to house amputees close together, if possible, for consistent nursing care and to allow patients to talk with and watch each other and to share their successes. Generally the postsurgical care of an amputee may also be thought of as the preprosthetic time when care goals by all team members focus on wound healing, limb and/or joint preparation, and early exercise, including ambulation. The specifics of each case may differ due to etiology, concomitant disease or trauma, age, motivation, and philosophy of the managing team.

The involvement of the physical therapist in the postoperative management of the below-knee amputee starts as soon as the amputee has been discontinued from any strong pain medication. The program can be much the same for all below-knee amputees, irrespective of the type of postoperative dressing used. Amputees usually come to the physical therapy department twice daily and are involved with an overall exercise program graded to each amputee's tolerance. Short periods of standing can reacquaint the amputee with balancing in the upright position. Mirrors are very helpful in providing visual feedback. Standing often occurs in a graded sequence, starting with bedside activity prior to coming to the physical therapy department. Initial standing may start on a tilt table to better control the body as well as blood pressure.

In addition to standing, amputees can begin doing quadriceps setting exercises, which are done every hour they are awake. This exercise increases strength and control of the quadriceps mechanism and can easily be done irrespective of the type of postoperative dressing applied. Progressive resistive exercise is usually discouraged due to the potential danger to the anterodistal-tibial skin closure. Skin problems are the primary reason for not wearing a prosthesis in below-knee amputees; therefore, great care should be exercised to keep the anterodistal tibia and tibial tubercular skin free of ulceration. Attention must also be given to the upper extremities, and progressive resistive exercise, using either diagonal patterns or conventional shoulder and elbow extension.

Soon after the amputee is able to stand comfortably and safely, he or she begins transfers. This enables the amputee to begin to care for himself or herself. Bed-to-chair, chair-to-commode, and chair-to-mat transfers are all important. During transfer and ambulation training, amputees fall often. Amputees who fall with a rigid dressing properly in place are less likely to injure the residual limb than with a soft dressing.

Once standing is safe and transfers are possible, one-legged hopping can be started. Hopping usually begins within the parallel bars and moves on to a walker and eventually crutches. Amputees usually do quite well with this phase but may expect too much from themselves too early. Very often amputees need to be told to rest, since they are eager to perform. If the amputee has been fitted with a plaster postsurgical dressing, it is imperative that the waist-belt suspension strap remain tight. Once the amputee is able to handle both the plaster and the walker, he or she is free to walk with assistance on the hospital unit, to encourage bed-to-toilet independence. Very often this independence coincides with the seventh to tenth postoperative day, at which time the sutures may be removed. However, many surgeons desire to leave sutures in much longer, particularly if wire has been used, since wire does not tend to cause problems with suture-line infections. On or around the 14th postoperative day, the sutures may be evaluated following removal of the first rigid dressing. Whether the sutures come out or not, another rigid dressing is applied and pylon added if the wound is healing satisfactorily.

If the amputee is placed in a soft dressing, stump wrapping begins in an effort to begin shrinking and shaping the residual limb. If possible, another member of the family is asked to share in the responsibility for stump wrapping. Diagrams illustrating the modified figure-of-eight method can be given to the amputee as a guide once the amputee leaves the hospital.

Use of a Temporary Prosthesis

The goals associated with the use of temporary prostheses include (1) independent ambulation; (2) independent donning and doffing; (3) understanding of socket fit; (4) understanding potential, excessive pressure areas; (5) learning who to call if problems arise. Most temporary prosthetic systems at the below-knee level allow the amputee to ambulate well independently while using a cane, crutch, or walker. Amputees should learn to walk with little assistance from others, unless balance or other problems persist. The temporary prosthetic device functions mostly as the definitive limb; it just does not have the cosmetic appearance of the finished limb.

Gait training begins in the parallel bars and progresses to whatever type of assistive device is mutually acceptable. Many amputees remain with a walker for some time. This is done to allow the stump to become conditioned by remaining in a partial weight-bearing situation. Amputees may be moved to forearm crutches, by choice, to enable them to load the prosthesis and to not lean on the axilla. In time, and in appropriate cases, amputees are encouraged to walk without any assistive devices. Typically amputees will take a long prosthetic step on the involved side, which makes equal step lengths difficult. A force plate can be used to make certain that the amputee is not overloading the new device.

Time must be spent teaching the amputee and family members about evaluating correct socket fit. Powder can be dusted into the socket and then examined after the stump is removed to determine if there has been total contact with the distal portions. Plastic temporary devices are often fabricated to fit over at least one 3-ply sock, which means that the chances of adding socks over the next three to six months are quite high. Care should be taken to instruct the patient in the correct socket fit. Measurements of circumferential changes should be taken at each follow-up visit, thus yielding an objective means of determining when the limb volume has stabilized and when it is time to fabricate the definitive device.

The Definitive Prosthesis

When the amputee is ready for the definitive fitting, another plaster impression or cast is taken. The socket is then mounted on the adjustable leg or jig and can be sent to the physical therapy department for gait evaluation and final changes, after which the device is returned to the prosthetist for definitive lamination. Experience has shown that this approach is more satisfactory than when the finished limb is delivered prior to any gait training or evaluation. These steps may seem time consuming for the prosthetist, but they ultimately save time by avoiding realignment after definitive lamination has occurred.

Amputees should learn to put on and take off the prosthesis with little assistance from others. The acceptance of any prosthesis depends a great deal on the ease with which the patient independently applies the device. It is the job of the physical therapist to teach the patient about the fit of the socket prior to discharge from the prosthetic training program. The understanding of the pressure and relief areas of the socket design will allow the amputee to continuously check the fit and to know when a stump sock must be added or removed. If the amputee is taught where excessive pressure areas are likely to develop, it is possible to troubleshoot problems at home. It is also important to discuss the difference between end bearing and total contact. Often it is beneficial to teach this same information to a significant other so that the amputee has another person to discuss these matters with in times of question. The last item necessary for the amputee is the name and phone number of someone to call if problems arise. In many cases this person(s) is a member of the prosthetic/orthotic clinic team and is likely to be the physical therapist. This gives the care a specialized touch and allows the amputee exact knowledge of who to contact if a question or problem arises.

ENERGY EXPENDITURE AND GAIT IN BELOW-KNEE AMPUTEES

As presented in Chapter 3, any "abnormal" gait pattern, whether associated with below-knee amputation or not, results in an increased energy requirement. Energy efficiency is also related to walking speed, body weight, and the disease states present, particularly vascular diseases that affect the heart, lungs, and the peripheral vessels, both arterial and venous. The presence of a major limb amputation represents yet another confounding variable. Although the literature is difficult to evaluate because of inconsistent methods and terms, certain conclusions can be drawn.

Waters et al[39] published what is probably the most quoted article dealing with below-knee amputation and energy expenditure. Waters et al[39] reported on a comparative study of the energy expenditure of normal subjects and below-knee amputees. Results indicated that the speed of walking of the vascular below-knee amputee was 41% less than normal, and that those vascular amputees expended 55% more energy at that speed when compared to normal. For comparison, traumatic below-knee amputees walked 13% slower than normal, using 25% more energy than normal. The average below-knee amputee walked 36% slower than normal, expending 41% more kcal/m/min. Gonzales et al[40] reported that the below-knee amputees in his study walked at 64.4 m/min, or 22% slower than normal but that the energy to walk at that speed was equal to normal. Ganguli et al[41] reported a speed of 50 m/min and an increase of 33% in energy expenditure. Reitemeyer[42] reported that unilateral below-knee amputees walked 60 m/min, using 28% more energy per unit of distance walked. Ralston[43] reported a below-knee walking speed of 48.8 m/min compared to normal nonamputees at 73.2 m/min. Ralston[43] also reported that energy expenditure per minute was equal for below-knee amputees and normal subjects when self-selected velocities were used. From these various studies there appears to be a consensus that below-knee amputees walk slower than normal, expending more energy than nonamputees. No study quantifies the specific contributions of length of residual limb, height, or the severity of the underlying peripheral vascular disease.

Du Bow et al[44] reported on six bilateral, dysvascular, below-knee amputees compared to eight nonamputee, age-matched controls. Both groups walked 40 m at a self-selected rate and exercised on a stationary ergometer. Results indicated that the controls walked 63 m/min, compared with 40 m/min for the amputees. The controls walked 48% faster than they propelled the ergometer (62.6 v 45.5 m/min). Oxygen consumption was 157% more for walking than for using a wheelchair. Bilateral below-knee amputees walked 39.9 m/min, or 1.5 mph, using 7.84 mL O_2/kg/min and 0.232 mL O_2/kg/m. Given the 39.9 m/min walking speed, this represents about half normal walking speed, with equal consumption and efficiency. Since energy to propel a wheelchair was 157% less than ambulation, it is easy to understand why bilateral amputees often choose a wheelchair.

Volpicelli et al[45] and Wagner[46] reviewed 44 cases of bilateral, below-knee amputation fitted with prostheses. Results indicated that 35 were rehabilitated, while nine were wheelchair ambulators. Twenty-three of 35 were defined as community ambulators, while 12 were household ambulators. Eighteen of 19 aged 60 years or less were rehabilitated, while only 17 of 25 aged 60 years or more were rehabilitated. Below-knee amputees from trauma did better than those with dysvascular diagnoses, and those not having major organic complications of diabetes did better than those who did. The data appeared to support the conclusion that bilateral Syme's or one below-knee and one Syme's did better than bilateral below-knee amputees. Although these numbers are quite small, several failures existed in these groups. However, the group with bilateral below-knee amputees were greater than 70 years of age and had major organ complications from diabetes. The results emphasize the importance of saving the knee joint but caution about the ultimate predictable success of rehabilitation with bilateral below-knee amputation and vascular disease. From these studies and others it has generally been concluded that the shorter the length of the below-knee stump the more energy consuming the gait.

Nielsen, Shurr, Goldman, and Meier[22] reported on seven traumatic below-knee amputations, comparing the energy cost using a conventional foot (SACH) and the Flex-Foot. Prior to this study research centered on the length of limb, age, or medical condition of the amputee, with little, if any, emphasis focused on prosthetic components. Seven amputees walked on a level treadmill at speeds ranging from 1.0 to 4.0 mph. (80 m/min = 3 mph). Although the number of subjects was small, several conclusions were warranted. Ambulation using the Flex-Foot facilitated a more normal walking speed (77.8 m/min) when amputees were allowed to select their own walking speed. Ambulation using the Flex-Foot at walking speeds greater than 2.5 mph (69 m/min) tended to conserve energy, on the average about 20% (mL/kg·m), resulting in lower relative levels of exercise intensity and enhanced gait efficiency.

REFERENCES

1. Wagner J, Supan T, Sienko S, Barth D. Motion analysis of SACH vs. Flex-Foot™ in moderately active below-knee amputees. *Clin Prosthet Orthot.* 1987; **11**(1):55–62.
2. LeBlanc MA. Elasti-liner type of Syme's prosthesis: Basic procedure and variation. *Artificial Limbs.* 1971; **15**:22–26.
3. Hornby R, Harris WR. Symes' amputation: Follow-up study of weight-bearing in 68 patients. *J Bone Joint Surg.* 1975; **57A**:346–349.
4. Davidson WH, Bohne WHO. The Syme amputation in children. *J Bone Joint Surg.* 1974; **56A**:1312.
5. Eilert RE, Jayakuram SS. *Boyd and Syme amputations in children. Jour Bone Joint Surg* 1976; **58A**:1138.
6. Sarmiento A, Gilmer RE, Finnieston A. A new surgical-prosthetic approach to the Syme's amputation: a preliminary report. *Art Limbs.* 1966; **10**:52–55.
7. Kay HW, Newman JD. Relative incidences of new amputations. *Orthot Prosthet.* 1975; **29**:3–16.
8. McCollough NC. The dysvascular amputee. *Orthop Clin North Am.* 1972; **3**(2):303–321.
9. Moore W, Hall AD, Wilie EJ. Below knee amputations for vascular insufficiency. *Arch Surg.* 1968; **97**:886.
10. Persson BM, Liedberg E. Measurement of maximal end-weight bearing in lower limb amputees. *Prosthet Orthot Int.* 1982; **6**:147–151.
11. Shea JD. Surgical techniques for lower extremity amputation. *Orthot Clin North Am.* 1972; **3**(2):287–301.
12. Tracy GD. Below knee amputation for ischemic gangrene. *Pac Med Surg.* 1966; **74**:251–253.
13. Persson BM. Sagittal incision for below knee amputation in ischemic gangrene. *J Bone Joint Surg.* 1974; **56B**:110–114.
14. Termansen WB. Below knee amputation for ischemic gangrene. *ACTA Orthop Scand.* 1977; **48**:311–316.

15. Burgess EM, Romano RL, Zettl JH, Schrock RD. Amputations of the leg for peripheral vascular insufficiency. *J Bone Joint Surg.* 1971; **53A**(5):874–890.

16. Burgess EM, Zettl JH. Amputations below the knee. *Art Limbs.* 1969; **13**(1):1–12.

17. Fishman S, Berger N, Watkins D. A survey of prosthetic practice—1973–74. *Orthot Prosthet.* 1975; **29**(3):15–20.

18. Lehneis HR. Prosthetics update 1980: Foot and knee components. *Newsletter: Prosthetics Orthotic* 1980, **4**(1):1–8.

19. Skinner HB, et al. Static load response of the heels of SACH feet. *Orthopedics.* 1985; **8**(2):225–228.

20. Doane N, Holt LE. A comparison of the SACH and single axis foot in the gait of unilateral below-knee amputees. *Prosthet Orthot Int.* 1983; **7**:33–36.

21. Burgess EM, et al. The Seattle foot—A design for active sports: Preliminary studies. *Orthot Prosthet.* Spring, 1983; **37**:25–31.

22. Nielsen DH, Shurr DG, Golden JC, Meier K. Comparison of energy cost and gait efficiency during ambulation in below-knee amputees using different prosthetic feet—a preliminary report. *J Prosthet Orthot.* 1988; **1**:24–31.

23. Koepke GH, Giacinto JP, McCumber RA. Silicone gel below-knee amputation prostheses. *Univ Mich Med Ctr J.* 1970; **36**:188–189.

24. Berlemont M, Weber R, Willot JP. Ten years of experience with the immediate application of prosthetic devices to amputees of the lower extremities on the operating table. *Prosthet Int.* 1969; **3**:8–18.

25. Mooney V, et al. Comparison of postoperative stump management: Plaster vs. soft dressings. *J Bone Joint Surg.* March, 1971; **53A**(2):241–249.

26. Baker WH, Barnes R, Shurr DG. The healing of below-knee amputations: A comparison of soft and plaster dressings. *Am J Surg.* 1977; **133**:716.

27. Isherwood PA, Robertson JC, Rossi A. Pressure measurements beneath below knee amputation stump bandages: Elastic bandaging the puddifoot dressing and a pneumatic bandaging technique compared *Br J Surg.* 1975; **62**:982–986.

28. Varghese G. Pressure applied by elastic prosthetic bandages: A comparative study. *Orthot Prosthet.* 1981; **35**:30–36.

29. Wu Y, Krick H. Removable rigid dressing for below-knee amputees. *Clin Prosthet Orthot.* 1987; **2**(1):34–44.

30. Gay R, Heard G. Long posterior flap below-knee amputation for obliterative vascular disease of the lower limb. *Int J Med Sci.* 1972; **141**(1–3):141–143.

31. Ghiulamila RI. Semirigid dressing for postoperative fitting of below-knee prosthesis. *Arch Phys Med Rehabil.* 1972; **53**:186–190.

32. Little JM. A pneumatic weight-bearing tempory prosthesis for below-knee amputees. *Lancet.* 1971; **1**:271–273.

33. Kerstein MD. Utilization of an air splint after below-knee amputation. *Am J Phys Med.* 1974; **53**(3):119–126.

34. Sher MH. The air splint. *Arch Surg.* 1974; **108**:746–747.

35. Silbert S. Amputation of the lower extremity in diabetes mellitus: Follow-up of 294 cases. *Diabetes.* 1952; **1**:297–299.

36. Mazet R. The geriatric amputee. *Art Limbs.* 1967; **11**:33–41.

37. Whitehouse FW, Jurgensen C, Block MA. The later life of the diabetic amputee: Another look at the fate of the second leg. *Diabetes.* 1968; **17**:520.

38. McCollough NC, Jennings JJ, Sarmiento A: Bilateral below the knee amputations in patients over fifty years of age. *J Bone Joint Surg.* 1972; **54A**(6):1217–1223.

39. Waters RL, Perry J, Antonelli D, Hislop H. Energy cost of walking of amputees: Influence of level of amputation. *J Bone Joint Surg.* 1976; **58**:42–46.

40. Gonzalez EG, Corcoran PJ, Reyes RL. Energy expenditure in below knee amputees: Correlation with stump length. *Arch Phys Med Rehabil.* 1974; **55**:111–119.

41. Ganguli S, Datta SR, Chatterjee BB, et al. Performance evaluation of amputee-prosthesis system in below-knee amputees. *Ergonomics.* 1973; **16**:797–810.

42. Reitemeyer H. Energieumsatz und Gangbild beim Gehen und Radfahren mit einem Unterschenkelkunstbein. *Z Orthop.* 1955; **86**:571–582.

43. Ralston HJ. Energy-speed relation and optimal speed during level walking. *Int Zeipschrife Angewandte Physiol Einschliesslich Aarbeitsphysiol.* 1958; **17**:277–283.

44. DuBow LL, Witt PL, Kadaba MP, Reyes R, Cochran GVB. Oxygen consumption of elderly persons with bilateral below knee amputations: Ambulation vs. wheelchair propulsion. *Arch Phys Med Rehabil.* 1983; **64**:255–259.

45. Volpicelli LJ, Chambers RB, Wagner FW. Ambulation levels of bilateral lower-extremity amputees. *J Bone Joint Surg.* 1983; **65A**(5):599–605.

46. Wagner FW. Amputations of the foot and ankle. *Clin Orthop.* 1977; **122**:62–69.

CHAPTER 5

Above-Knee Amputations and Prostheses

Above-knee amputations, although not as common as below-knee amputations, are done for the very same medical reasons as below-knee amputations, namely, trauma, tumor, disease, and congenital defects. Unfortunately, primary bone tumors often affect the proximal bone of the extremities and often the more proximal joints. According to Aitken,[1] of 136 amputations performed for tumors of the lower extremity, all but eight were done at the level of the knee disarticulation or higher, and 48 required either hip disarticulation of hemipelvectomy. Although greater than 80% of all amputations are done for vascular reasons,[2] the occurrence of above-knee amputation was reported to be 44.1% in 1964 but only 32.6% in 1975. The percentage is probably reduced even further today. According to the most recent data,[2] 84.9% of all above-knee amputations occur between the ages of 50 and 80 years. Congenital amputations and limb deficiencies will be discussed in Chapter 8.

As a general rule, the shorter the amputated limb above the knee, the less satisfactory the functional outcome and the less likely the amputee may be to continue to use an artificial limb. McCollough et al[3] reported that only 45% of above-knee amputees over 50 years of age can expect to ambulate using an above-knee prosthesis, and only 30% who are over 55 years of age can expect to ambulate. Since there is general recognition that this situation exists, surgeons attempt to save the knee joint whenever possible.

Given this rather bleak picture, it becomes the goal of the clinic team to attempt to provide prostheses to only those above-knee amputees who can be reasonably expected to use them successfully. Unfortunately, this decision-making process in not easy and clear-cut; much success is due to trial and error and to the expertise of a knowledgeable and experienced health care team.

This chapter will describe above-knee amputation and prosthetic levels, along with prosthetic components. Suspension of above-knee prostheses and considerations for managing the residual limb will then be presented. Finally, alignment of above-knee prostheses will be discussed along with training the amputee to become a functional prosthetic user. A section is also included on knee disarticulation.

LEVELS OF ABOVE-KNEE AMPUTATION

The term above-knee amputation, for the purposes of this chapter, will include all amputation and prosthetic levels from knee disarticulation up to hip disarticulation and hemipelvectomy. It should be kept in mind, however, that the vast majority of above-knee amputations occurs at approximately the midthigh level (Fig. 5–1).

Knee Disarticulation (Through Knee)

The knee disarticulation, or through-knee amputation, is a level not often seen in America. Most support for this level comes from European and, particularly, British literature. In the older population, the through-knee level is said to offer an advantage, since side-to-side flaps are thought to enhance wound healing. For those individuals who are not likely to be functional ambulators, this level is thought to offer the mechanical advantage of a longer lever arm for greater ease in transfers and related activities.

Shea[4] states that the through-knee amputation offers an end-bearing residual limb with increased proprioception as compared to other levels. In addition to affording

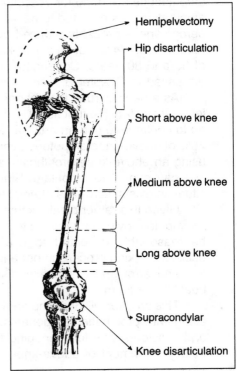

Figure 5–1. Levels of above-knee amputation. (From Northwestern University Prosthetic Orthotic Center, with permission, 1987.)

excellent prospects for suspension of the prosthesis, it is a relatively easy surgical procedure to carry out and is quite safe for the patient. However, Shea[4] also believes that a primary knee disarticulation should not occur if the patient has a preexisting hip-flexion contracture.

Knee disarticulation is a level often considered for growing children, since it preserves the distal femoral epiphysis and allows distal femoral growth to continue following the amputation. In children the level is often end bearing and does not require a socket design that unloads the limb proximally.

Above-Knee Amputation

Since most above-knee amputations are performed for vascular reasons, the procedure can be considered to be elective, that is, done in a nonemergent situation and at an anatomic level of the surgeon's choosing. This situation allows the surgeon to consult with the prosthetist and physical therapist if questions arise as to the ideal functional prosthetic level.

Although the surgical procedure involved in performing an above-knee level amputation may not require a great deal of technical skill, Mooney[5] cautions that several important considerations must be taken into account before making the decision to operate. If the amputee is a likely candidate for a prosthesis, a more technical procedure must be accomplished to allow the amputee the best chance of prosthetic and rehabilitative success.

The problem with primary wound healing at the above-knee level is not nearly as great as with the below-knee level. In fact, amputation at the above-knee level was the most prevalent lower-limb amputation for many years because of predictable wound healing. Much has been written concerning the subject of muscle stabilization in the above-knee amputation. There was a time when myodesis, or the surgical securing of the muscle to the bone, was advocated by many authorities. Today, myoplasty is thought to be sufficient. This involves trimming the muscles and suturing them into the respective fascia, anterior muscles on the front and posterior muscles on the back. This prevents the residual limb and especially the proximal thigh from altering shape after the prosthetic socket has been fabricated.

Long Above-Knee Amputation. The long above-knee amputation may be thought of as being supracondylar, that is, the length of the femur extends down as far as the condyles. The supracondylar level produces a long and effective lever arm with which to control the prosthesis. All hip musculature is left intact and available to control the prosthesis. As long as the hip extensors and abductors are not altered, the prosthetic gait expectation should be excellent. A long, residual limb with all normal motion and musculature allows both the patient and the prosthetist the freedom to use a variety of components, not being hampered by a stump that is too long or too short by a lack of muscular control. It also allows for "standard" alignment of the limb.

"Standard" Above-Knee Amputation. The medium length, or "standard," above-knee amputation may be considered as midthigh in length, bisecting the femur. In many cases this level allows the use of standard above-knee components and results in good gait. Although all muscle groups are intact at this level, it is important to realize that the higher up the amputation occurs, the greater the pressure on the socket, especially the lateral aspects. At this level a long anterior flap is often used to avoid having the suture line on the bottom of the socket.

Short Above-Knee Amputation. The short above-knee level is generally thought to be 5 to 7 cm in length. At this level the short length of the residual limb makes stabilization of the hip in stance phase quite difficult. Suspension of the limb also becomes more of a problem the more proximal the amputation, since there is less tissue to grasp. Since some weight bearing occurs on the posterior soft tissue of the thigh, the shorter the thigh the less available surface area. With a short above-knee stump, the ability of the thigh to generate forces to control the knee during both swing and stance is reduced and provides limitations on the type of knee unit that can be used in the prosthesis. Amputation at the short above-knee level also increases the chances of muscle imbalance, where the hip flexors overpower the hip extensors, resulting in a hip-flexion contracture. Abduction and external rotation may also be present.

A very short above-knee amputation may occur at the level of the lesser trochanter of the femur or more proximally. The potential problems that were just discussed become even more pronounced with a very short stump. Mechanically the very small lever is quite ineffective in controlling a standard above-knee prosthesis. Much pressure is taken on the lateral distal femur in an attempt to stabilize the hip mediolaterally in stance phase. Suspension at this level can also be difficult. It may not be possible to use certain suspension techniques, and the amputee needs to be cautioned that the limb may lose suspension at inopportune times. It is not uncommon for an amputee in a quadrilateral socket with a very short stump to actually come out of the prosthesis when sitting in a chair.

COMPONENTS OF ABOVE-KNEE PROSTHESES

Components unique to prostheses at the knee disarticulation level are discussed at the end of this chapter. The following section discusses components used for a typical above-knee prosthesis (designed to accommodate an amputation at the approximate midthigh level). Four major components can be identified: the prosthetic foot, spacer, knee unit, and above-knee socket.

Above-Knee Prosthetic Foot

Prosthetic feet used in above-knee prostheses are the same as those used in below-knee prostheses. Because of greater concern for the knee than for the ankle/foot, the vast majority of prosthetic feet used in above-knee prosthetics today are solid-ankle–cushion-heel (SACH) prosthetic feet because of their simplicity and dependability.

Above-Knee Prosthesis Spacers

The basic structure of an above-knee prosthesis can be provided by either an endoskeletal or exoskeletal system, essentially identical to those used in below-knee prostheses.

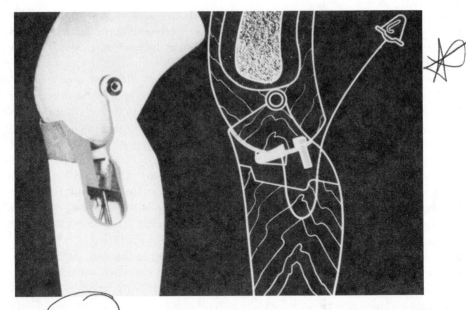

Figure 5–2. Locked knee, also called a positive locked knee. Amputee pulls cord to unlock knee, an internal spring locks knee when knee is initially extended. (From Otto Bock, Orthopedic Industry, Inc. Minneapolis, MN, with permission.)

Above-Knee Prosthetic Knees

Ideally a prosthetic knee unit substitutes for the normal knee functions of shock absorption and support during stance phase and swing-phase flexion during gait. Realistically, as with prosthetic feet, compromises in function must be accepted. Numerous knee units are available for above-knee prostheses and may be thought of as occurring in a functional continuum from a simple locked knee to a relatively sophisticated, hydraulically controlled unit designed to provide control during both swing and stance phase of gait.

The Locked Knee. A locked knee allows no swing-phase knee flexion and provides complete stability in stance phase. Typical examples of locked-knee prostheses are shown in Figure 5–2 and range from a peg leg having a wooden or metal pipe with no articulation to standard locked-knee units made by Otto Bock and others to ensure knee stability primarily for the geriatric amputee.

Clinically the prosthetic team needs to make a decision based on the individual needs of the amputee as to whether or not to recommend a locked knee. Very often, in the early phases of gait training with the dysvascular amputee and one whom the team is not certain will be a successful prosthetic user, a simple locked-knee pipe or pylon may be used. This allows for a quick evaluation of the amputee's abilities and still allows the amputee to unlock and bend the knee while sitting. It is not uncommon for a definitive above-knee prosthesis for a geriatric patient to contain a locked knee. Typically these prostheses use knee units that have spring assists that lock when the amputee straightens the knee in extension. Flexion of the knee is produced by pulling a cord attached to the lateral socket just before sitting. It is important to remember that the absence of knee flexion in swing phase will necessitate some other changes in the prosthesis, often shortening of the overall length. Such shortening will allow for swing phase on the prosthetic side without marked circumduction, hip hiking, or vaulting, all energy-consuming gait deviations. Using a simple locked-knee unit, a definitive above-knee prosthesis may be made completely from plastic, so the overall weight of the device may be less than 5 lb.

Single-Axis, Constant-Friction Knee. The single-axis (SA), constant-friction knee unit is a common choice. As the name implies, friction in the knee unit remains constant throughout the gait cycle. The SA knee allows flexion and extension, and the constant friction control limits the speed of the motion. Typically the friction is produced by a mechanical collar around the knee axis, having screw controls that affect the tightness of the collar and therefore the amount of friction applied to the axis. The screws, usually two in number, are located on the posterior side of the knee unit, analogous to the popliteal space. The adjustment of these screws limits the speed at which the amputee may walk and also somewhat limits the amount of knee flexion or heel rise generated by the prosthesis during swing phase. Figure 5–3 shows a typical SA constant-friction knee unit.

Stance phase stability is provided principally by the alignment of the knee unit within the prosthesis. This type of knee unit is often used with amputees having medium to long stumps who achieve stance-phase knee stability by having a posteriorly offset knee axis and who achieve swing-phase control from constant friction. The SA,

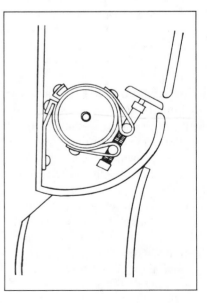

Figure 5–3. The SA, constant-friction knee component. Lateral view of a single axis constant friction knee.

constant-friction knee also may be used in children whose overall height is very small and in whom no sophisticated knee-control mechanism is usually necessary.

Theoretically an amputee will carry around a screwdriver and change the amount of friction depending upon the desired speed of walking. Realistically this does not occur, as most amputees set the friction control at a speed suitable for most of their activities and rarely, if every, change it until a new prosthesis is necessary.

"Locking"-Knee (Weight-Activated Stance Control). Another major type of above-knee prosthetic knee unit is referred to as a locking knee. Locking knees function as a SA knee during swing and as a locked knee during stance. Most locking knees will lock as an axial load is applied following foot contact and will remain locked until the weight has been shifted to the sound side after heel off, just before toe off. At this point the initiation of knee flexion in swing phase is begun, and the prosthesis acts as any normal SA knee.

Probably the best known member of this group of prosthetic knees is the wooden exoskeletal version of the Otto Bock safety knee (Fig. 5–4). This safety knee consists of two pieces of wood wedged in the shape of a "V" to accommodate one another. Upon loading, the wedges come together, creating friction between the wooden components and rendering the knee locked. Upon the weight transfer to the sound side, a spring separates the two wedges, and the knee functions as any other SA, constant-friction unit. During swing phase the Bock safety knee has constant-friction screw adjustments in the posterior popliteal area. As can be seen in Figure 5–4, the Bock safety knee also has a round plastic wheel (gait-regulator screw) that should not be confused in function

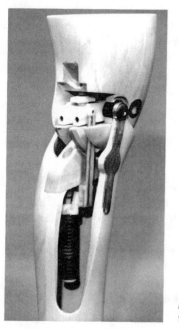

Figure 5–4. Otto Bock weight-activated lock (safety knee): knee in the exoskeletal version.

with the friction-adjustment screws. The wheel allows for approximation of the wooden components as the surfaces wear down, while the screws are responsible for the amount of constant friction in the knee. It is not uncommon for patients and therapists to confuse the purposes of these two adjustments and to use the approximation function as a means of swing-phase control that prematurely wears out the wooden components. The anterior view of the Bock safety knee also shows a rubber extension stop that is responsible for maintaining the knee in neutral and not allowing it to hyperextend. Patients may sometimes remove the rubber anterior stop to place the device in hyperextension, making the knee joint very stable. This should be discouraged, as it prematurely wears out the knee. Properly adjusted and used, the safety knee requires very little maintenance, is durable in all types of weather and occupations, and is generally considered to be one of the most reliable knee joints available.

The Bock safety knee is also available in the endoskeletal model, operating from a slightly different design but clinically delivering very similar function. The safety knees as a group afford the amputee the safety and peace of mind of having inherent knee stability in stance phase and freedom of knee flexion in swing phase without spring-loaded locks or releases that need to be activated by the patient prior to sitting. This knee unit does not allow an amputee to flex the prosthetic knee while going down a ramp or stairs, since weight application to the device locks it at that point. This fact needs to be kept in mind when prescribing a prosthesis that includes a safety knee. The necessity to walk on uneven surfaces such as rough ground or gravel often is considered an indication for the safety knee, since the knee locks when weight is applied in stance phase irrespective of the position of the hip, the force exerted by the hip, or the position of the foot and ankle. The Bock safety knee will also lock at other-than-complete extension; thus, in the case of an incomplete step the prosthetic knee will be locked 10 to 15 degrees short of extension just as well as in full extension. This allows the amputee a small margin of error in swing phase so that if during terminal deceleration of the shank the heel hits the floor before full knee extension, the prosthetic knee will still be locked and the patient will not stumble.

Recently a French company, Proteor, introduced a modification of the locking knee. It is very similar to the Otto Bock endoskeletal knee, having the ability to lock in any position of prosthetic knee flexion. This feature allows the knee to lock in those situations in which it does not come to complete terminal extension and where some other locking knees would buckle. The knee is compatible with other endoskeletal systems.

Polycentric Knees. Greene[6] defines a polycentric knee as any knee designed to allow the shin to move in a combination of rotational and translational motion about an instantaneous center of rotation. Four-bar knees contain four elements, or arms, connected at four separate points. Because of the different lengths and attachments of these elements, the shin moves through a "polycentric" pattern as the knee flexes.

Greene[6] describes the characteristics of a four-bar knee using alpha and beta values. The alpha value is the distance that the instant center of rotation (ICR) is posterior to the trochanter-knee-ankle (TKA) line (to be described in a following section). The farther posterior the point of intersection of the two links of the knee, the more stable the knee. The beta value describes the distance from the ICR to the end of the residual limb. The more superior the ICR, the less flexion moment and the better the control of the knee.

Fluid Swing-Phase Control. Fluids, both oil and air, are used in cylinders in prosthetic knee units to control motion of the knee during the swing phase of gait (Fig. 5–5). Uneven or increased heel rise presents a problem for some amputees, since it increases the time needed for the swing phase, making it more difficult to have the limb on the floor ready to accept weight for the next stance phase. The faster the amputee walks, the more excessive the heel rise becomes, even though the time available to complete the swing phase is less at faster walking speeds. Swing-phase fluid-control devices are intended to minimize excessive heel rise and to provide resistance to knee motion that is proportional to walking speed. The resistance to knee flexion in swing phase is produced as the piston in the cylinder pushes against air or oil, depending on whether the system is pneumatic or hydraulic. The resistance of the swing triggers a knee extension bias that then assists the prosthetic knee into extension. These systems are adjustable in the sense that the knee extension bias may be adjusted by the prosthetist, therapist, or patient in an effort to minimize the time spent in knee flexion and to maximize the angle near extension so that faster gaits can be optimized.

Most, but not all, systems with hydraulic or pneumatic swing-phase control cylinders have no adjustable mechanism to provide stability in stance. Therefore all control of stance phase is achieved by alignment and by muscular contraction of the hip extensors during stance phase.

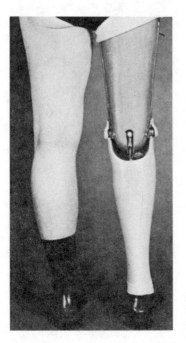

Figure 5–5. Fluid swing-phase control knee unit. (From Wilson AB. Recent advances in AK prostheses. *Art Limbs*. 1968; **12**:14, with permission.)

The indications for use of a hydraulic or pneumatic swing-phase control unit are generally thought to be related directly to the functional abilities or desires of the amputee. Unless the amputee desires a variable cadence, it probably is not necessary to use fluid swing-phase control mechanism. Generally the longer the above-knee residual limb the greater the flexion force at the hip that can be generated, and the greater the resultant knee flexion during swing phase. If this amount of knee flexion presents a problem, a swing-phase control mechanism like the fluid control devices might be considered.

It is important to realize that the addition of a fluid swing-phase control mechanism adds not only weight but also expense to the prosthesis. It is therefore often unwise to add these devices to the prostheses of elderly, less active amputees.

Swing- and Stance-Phase Fluid Control. On the far end of the continuum of knee units for above-knee prostheses are the devices that provide fluid control of both swing and stance phase. The devices described to this point have all been examples of cadence-dependent devices, that is, the settings of either the adjustment screws, or valves in the case of fluid control devices, were relative to a specific desired gait speed, and further adjustments were needed if the amputee made significant changes in walking speed. Figure 5–6 represents the most sophisticated above-knee component

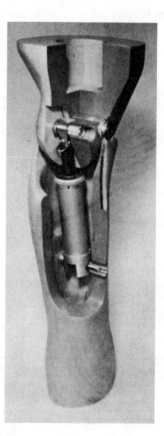

Figure 5–6. The Mauch SNS Swing and Stance fluid control knee unit.

currently available. It contains hydraulic swing- and stance-phase control mechanism that is considered to function independently of walking cadence, giving the amputee the ability to run one step and to walk the next, adjusting to whatever cadence the amputee desires on a step-by-step basis. This feature clearly separates this swing- and stance-phase fluid control (SNS) device from all others.

The stance-phase component allows the amputee to walk down stairs or ramps step over step. Since the knee does not lock, as in the case of the locking knee, or stay locked, as in the case of the locked knee, the fluid-controlled stance-phase mechanism allows a gradual yielding of the knee from extension to flexion with the rate depending upon the amount of weight applied to the limb at that particular setting. This gradual knee flexion allows the amputee to essentially "ride" the hydraulic cylinder down the steps one at a time and to follow the prosthetic step with a normal step on the sound side. This does away with the necessity for walking down stairs one step at a time, turning sideways, or experiencing what is referred to as "jackknifing" to descend stairs or ramps.

The swing-phase control portion of the SNS unit functions very similarly to other commercially available fluid-control systems except that it requires a hyperextension moment at heel off and during toe off to initiate knee flexion in swing phase. This is an important learning consideration for any amputee who might be switching from a less sophisticated knee unit to an SNS unit. This knee hyperextension maneuver is also necessary prior to the amputee's sitting in a chair. To accomplish this the amputee must stand before the chair with the prosthetic leg behind the sound leg; apply a force through the toe of the prosthesis, hyperextending the knee; and then quickly flex the hip and knee to sit on the chair. If the extension moment is not generated just before attempting to sit, the knee stance-phase control will remain in effect, and the time from standing to sitting will be slowed to allow for the graded yielding of the knee as it would in any other situation.

There are situations in which the amputee may wish to take the stance-phase control mode off completely. To accomplish this the amputee must only stand with weight on the toe of the prosthesis and, while generating an extension moment, move the u-shaped lever on the posterior side of the device.

A third mode option locks the knee in a fixed flexion or extension position. To accomplish this the amputee flips the selector switch while a flexion moment exists. This is used, for instance, while driving a car.

Use of Knee Components. The "Newsletter" of the Prosthetic and Orthotics Clinic[7] surveyed prosthetics practitioners in 1980 to determine which prosthetic knees were most often used in the delivery of above-knee prostheses. It was reported that locking knees were used 27% of the time, safety knees 39%, constant-friction knees 12%, and hydraulic knees 8%. Therefore 66% of the knees delivered were either manual locking or safety knees.

Quadrilateral Socket

The quadrilateral socket for above-knee prostheses was designed by Radcliffe and Foort at the University of California at Berkeley in the early 1960s and is used almost universally in the United States today.[8] The quadrilateral socket was a departure from its predecessor, the "plug" socket, which was made of wood and was basically an ischial ring into which the amputee placed the residual limb.

As with the PTB socket for below-knee prostheses, the modern quadrilateral (or quad) socket is made of plastic laminate formed over a modified positive-plaster model of the residual limb. Likewise, the quadrilateral socket is intended to provide total contact but not end bearing. This means that the total contact at the bottom of the socket aids in the reduction of distal edema by not allowing the edema adequate space to exist. This feature of the socket keeps the volume of the distal residual limb constant. Additionally, it does not allow hard edema or induration, which may cause permanent changes in the appearance of the distal residual limb and produce the painful condition known as verrucous hyperplasia, as shown in Figure 5–7. A well-fitted quadrilateral socket will prevent this thickening of the skin.

As the name implies, the quadrilateral socket consists of four walls (Fig. 5–8). These are referred to as the anterior, posterior, medial, and lateral walls. Each wall has specific functions.

Posterior Wall. The top of the posterior wall, about 1 in lateral to the posteromedial corner, provides the main area of weight bearing for the ischial tuberosity. The location of the ischial tuborosity indicates whether the amputee is down into the socket proper-ly. To a lesser extent, the top of the posterior wall lateral to the ischial tuberosity also provides an area of some weight bearing for the gluteus maximus. The top edge of the

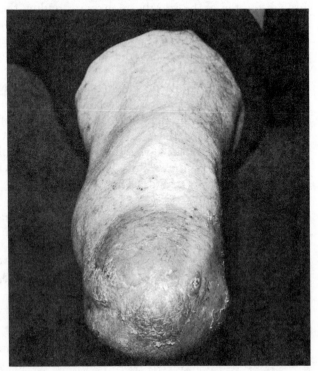

Figure 5–7. Verrucous hyperplasia due to inadequate total contact.

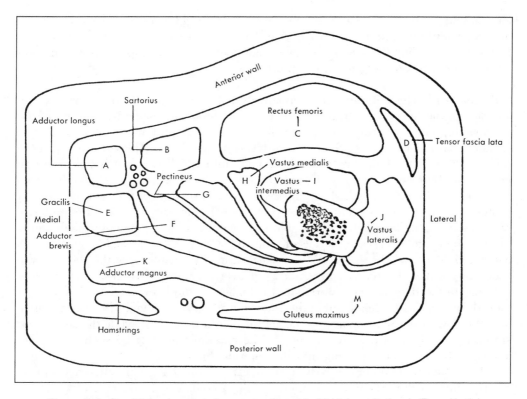

Figure 5–8. Quadrilateral socket. A cross-section at ischial tuberosity level. (From Northwestern University Prosthetic Orthotic Center, with permission, 1987.)

posterior wall is usually horizontal when the amputee is in single-limb support during gait. Many amputees are unable to tolerate a sharp-cornered shelf on which the ischial tuberosity sits so this portion of the posterior wall may need to be slightly rounded or modified to accommodate the shape of the gluteus maximus, depending on the individual. Slight modifications allow for more amputee comfort, without any loss of control.

Below the ischial seat the flat posterior wall provides a site against which the femur can exert posteriorly directed hip-extension moments. Depending on the experience and the philosophy of the prosthetist, the posterior wall may slope downward from back to front. This slope allows the posterior structures to better fit into the socket, causing them to be loaded more gradually.

As the posterior wall proceeds laterally, the width becomes less, to accommodate the gluteus maximus musculature. The angle created by the junction of the posterior and lateral walls will not always be 90 degrees but will depend somewhat on the bulk of the lateral musculature.

The presence of pain or burning on the posterior wall in the early days of initial gait training may not indicate a fault in prosthetic design or fabrication. Since the ischial tuberosity is only covered with periosteum and little, if any, muscle, the early days of gait training involve the bruising of the periosteum. This normally takes about three or four days to remedy. The complaint should be monitored for several days, as pain will not occur until the amputee is fully loading the posterior wall. Only then will the pain begin, thus signaling the start of dynamic alignment, since the amputee is now placing all of his or her body weight on the prosthesis.

Anterior Wall. The anterior wall is relatively flat and is shaped to conform to the anatomy of the femoral (or Scarpa's) triangle. The femoral triangle is made up of the inguinal ligament, the medial border of the sartorius, and the medial border of the adductor longus muscle. Since the sartorius muscle may be hypertrophied, there tends to be a slight indentation in the triangle into which the prosthetist places an appropriate bulge of the socket. The location of the femoral triangle is directly across from the location of the ischial tuberosity, allowing pressure in this area to create a posteriorly directed force tending to keep the ischial tuberosity on top of the posterior wall. Although the prosthetist is not able to heavily "load" the femoral triangle, force may be applied to this area of the socket. The height of the anterior wall in most cases is about 2.5 in above the level of the ischial seat. By maintaining this height, the posteriorly directed force can be spread out over a greater area, resulting in lower pressure to the tissues. The anterior wall is higher on the lateral side and drops as it joins the medial wall. The height of the anterior wall may be judged when the amputee sits. If the wall does not impinge on the anterosuperior iliac spine while the amputee is sitting in a chair, it is the proper height. The anterior wall may be slightly rounded anteriorly to avoid any pinching into the anterior thigh.

It is not uncommon in the early stages of gait training for the amputee to complain of discomfort in the region of the anterior wall. A common misconception is that the problem can be eliminated by "lowering" the anterior wall. However, reducing the height of the anterior wall will only make the problem worse, since it is the sole mechanism for maintaining the ischial tuberosity on the posterior wall. Removing this counter force allows the posterior structures to move anteriorly and in some cases to "fall inside" the socket, creating painful burning in the anteromedial corner.

Medial Wall. The medial wall of the quad socket contains the soft tissue of the medial thigh. The medial wall of the socket should be parallel to the amputee's line of progression or the direction in which the amputee is walking. The top edge of the medial wall may be angled downward, back to front, and may be one-half inch lower than the anterior wall to allow for clearance of the public ramus. The thickness of the medial wall is of concern, since a very thin medial wall can act as a knife blade, cutting the amputee with every step.

An important anatomic relief for the adductor longus tendon is placed in the anteromedial corner of the socket. This channel represents an important landmark for indicating whether the prosthesis is applied in the proper amount of rotation. Excess tissue not pulled inside the medial wall of the socket is referred to as an adductor roll. In addition to being painful, the presence of an adductor roll can limit the fit of the medial portion of the socket. Adductor rolls can be reduced by using compression wraps and may require this treatment indefinitely when the prosthesis is not being worn.

Lateral Wall. The function of the lateral wall is to provide a surface against which the lateral femur may push to stabilize the hip in stance phase. This lateral force of the femur is responsible for the mediolateral stability of the pelvis. As with any lever system, the longer the lever arm the greater the moment that can be generated and the less pressure that results. Therefore a shorter residual limb may have a higher lateral wall in an effort to provide enough surface area for stability.

Since the lateral wall meets the anterior wall in the anterolateral corner, the height of both walls of that point will be equal. The lateral wall is often curved to accommodate the shape of the tensor fascia lata. It proceeds posteriorly and joins the posterior wall, always remaining higher than the posterior wall.

Distally the lateral wall must accommodate the cut end of the femur, as direct pressure on the cut end of the bone is not well tolerated. It is not uncommon for the prosthetist to provide a built-up area just proximal to the end of the femur, where pressure can be better tolerated. The slope of the lateral wall determines the angle of preadduction, as explained in a following section.

Flexible Sockets

Although the vast majority of both below-knee and above-knee prosthetic sockets are made of hard plastic laminate, there has been recent interest in the development of sockets made of more flexible materials such as low-density polyethylene. Breakey[9] published an article in 1970 on the use of the flexible socket in the below-knee amputee. About 1975, Kristinsson,[10] a prosthetist from Reykjavik, Iceland, developed a flexible socket for a bilateral above-knee amputee who was not satisfied with the hard sockets that had been made for him. Since that time the emergence of new materials has allowed prosthetists many opportunities to experiment with new designs, attempting to improve the function and comfort of the socket on the amputee. Figure 5–9 shows a Scandinavian flexible socket. The socket is made of low-density polyethylene, while the brim is made of harder plastic laminate. The brim provides the structure necessary to transmit forces to and through the prosthetic limb, without affecting the flexibility of the socket.

Although no formal evaluation of these new sockets has been published, they are thought to provide the following improvements on conventional sockets: (1) less confining and therefore more comfortable; (2) better suspension due to the flexible material; (3) better proprioception; (4) cooler in hot weather.

New Socket Designs

A recent development in above-knee sockets is the concept of using a narrow mediolateral dimension, a larger anteroposterior dimension, and an increased adduction posture. Proponents of this "narrow M-L" system cite problems with current quad-socket technology.

These designs, developed from the basic work of Ivan Long, are currently in use in the United States and Europe. Problems associated with this new design are many, not the least of which involves teaching its use without follow-up clinical studies supporting it as a superior system to the quad socket.

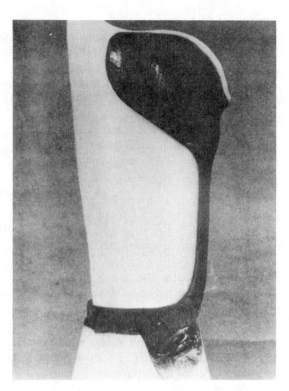

Figure 5–9. The Scandinavian flexible socket; above-knee level with rigid housing.

Preflexion of the Above-Knee Socket

In the discussion of the alignment of the below-knee prosthesis, the concept of preflexion was introduced. In the above-knee prosthesis a similar concept is used to preflex the quad socket prior to initial fitting and gait training. Preflexion of the above-knee socket is thought to increase prosthetic function in two ways. First, it allows easier access to the ischial tuberosity so that weight bearing may occur on the top edge of the posterior wall on and around the ischial tuberosity. The second objective of preflexion is to place the hip extensors in a somewhat stretched condition, enabling them to more powerfully extend the hip and to stabilize both the pelvis and the artificial knee during weight bearing. The preflexing of the above-knee socket also allows the amputee to walk with a more normal step length on the uninvolved, sound side.

For the prosthetist to determine the amount of initial or preflexion necessary, measurement of the amputee's hip range of motion in extension must be accomplished using the Thomas maneuver. The prosthetist will add 5 to 7 degrees of flexion to the socket in excess of the amputee's normal extension range of motion. That is, if an amputee can extend his or her amputated hip to neutral, the prosthetist will place the socket in 5 to 7 degrees of initial flexion. If an amputee has a 5-degree flexion contracture on the amputated side, then the prosthetist will place the socket into 10 to 12 degrees of initial flexion within the prosthesis. Once this preflexion has been built into the prosthesis and the amputee extends to the limits of his or her anatomic range of

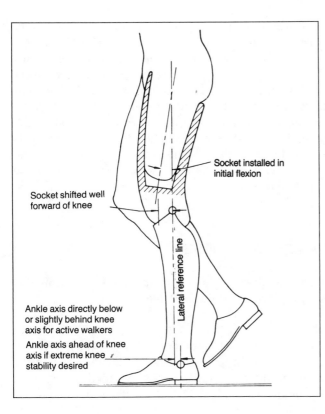

Socket installed in
initial flexion

Socket shifted well
forward of knee

Lateral reference line

Ankle axis directly below
or slightly behind knee
axis for active walkers

Ankle axis ahead of knee
axis if extreme knee
stability desired

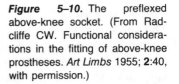

Figure   5–10. The   preflexed
above-knee socket. (From Radcliffe CW. Functional considerations in the fitting of above-knee
prostheses. *Art Limbs* 1955; **2**:40,
with permission.)

motion, the prosthesis will be in the degree of extension needed at the time of heel off
during gait (Fig. 5–10).

The presence or absence of the proper amount of initial flexion may be evidenced
by the degree to which the amputee exhibits lordosis, since insufficient preflexion of the
above-knee socket will require the amputee to compensate for inadequate extension of
the hip by rotating the pelvis and causing lordosis of the lumbar spine at the time to heel
off. In contrast, too much preflexion of the socket will produce difficulty in stabilizing
the prosthetic knee during the stance phase.

The appearance of the finished or definitive above-knee prosthesis may not clearly
show the amount of preflexion of the socket. In Figure 5–10 the line indicates the
orientation of a preflexed socket within a double-walled, above-knee, finished prosthesis. As can be seen, the socket can be substantially preflexed while the prosthesis
gives the overall appearance of being either in neutral or slightly extended. However,
limitations exist in excess of 25 degrees, since knee-center placement requirements may
make the device unacceptable cosmetically.

Preadduction of the Above-Knee Socket

As with preflexion of the above-knee socket, the prosthetist also preadducts the socket
prior to initial fitting and gait training. The purpose of preadducting the socket is to
place the hip abductors on slight stretch, allowing them to more forcefully abduct and

contribute to the overall stability of the hip on the amputated side in stance phase. Prosthetists are taught to preadduct above-knee sockets approximately 5 to 11 degrees, depending on the patient evaluation. This means that if the amputee has normal abduction and adduction of the hip, the socket will be placed in approximately 5 to 11 degrees of adduction greater than neutral. As will be described in the alignment section, the degree of preadduction in the socket depends on the overall length of the residual limb. The longer the residual limb, the more necessary it is to adduct the socket so that the centers of the heels are close together. The prosthetist preadducts the socket less the shorter the residual limb. This adduction concept differentiates the newer narrow M-L socket concepts from that of the quad socket. Since the normal adduction angle of the femur is physiologic as well as anatomic, the developers of the new designs stress adduction.

SUSPENSION OF ABOVE-KNEE PROSTHESES

There are three main systems for suspending an above-knee prosthesis: (1) a Silesian band or bandage, (2) a hip joint and pelvic band, and (3) suction.

Silesian Band

The Silesian band or bandages is comprised of a strap that originates on the lateral wall proximally and encircles the sound side of the pelvis, anchoring on the front of the socket with a buckle (Fig. 5–11). The Silesian band is usually intended to be only a suspension device, but, depending on the origination of the strap, it may assist in rotary control of the prosthesis in stance phase.

When this suspension is insufficient and if the prosthetist desires not to use another, more restrictive form of suspension, an auxiliary strap may be added to the Silesian band. This auxiliary strap originates on the back of the Silesian band and crosses up and over the hip on the amputated side, fastening to the anterior strap by means of a small buckle. The length of the residual limb usually dictates the need for an auxiliary strap. A very short residual limb does not have as much surface area; thus there may be a need for more suspension. It is possible, however, to use a Silesian band suspension in cases of very short amputations, particularly those done for primary bone tumors in children or young adults, where extra hardware is not desired. In one case the authors have successfully used Silesian band suspension with a residual limb amputated just above the lesser trochanter.

Hip Joint and Pelvic Band

If there is a need for more extensive suspension or if there is a need for increasing the effective height of the lateral wall to assist the hip in lateral stability, a hip joint and pelvic band may be indicated (Fig. 5–12). The need for improved hip stability in stance phase may result from either weak abductors or a short residual limb. By using the hip joint and pelvic band, the lateral wall is essentially lengthened, and the amount of muscle force required to stabilize the hip in stance phase is lessened. The amputee may actually lean into the hip joint in midstance, limiting the tendency to lean or list to the amputated side.

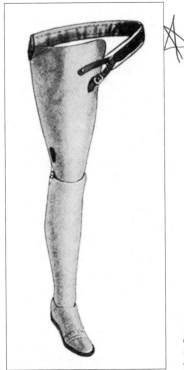

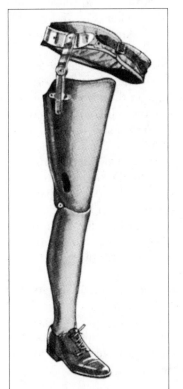

Figure 5–11. Silesian band suspension of above-knee prosthesis. (From Wilson AB. Limb prosthetics—1970. *Art Limbs.* 1970; **14**:31, with permission.)

Figure 5–12. Hip joint and pelvic band. (From Wilson AB. Limb prosthetics—1970. *Art Limbs.* 1970; **14**:31, with permission.

Although the use of a hip joint and pelvic band may sound like a complete system, the pelvic band or belt can hinder the amputee in sitting because of the single axis hip joint. If the hip joint is properly aligned for standing, it may not be so aligned for sitting, creating an internally rotated prosthetic limb and a problem with cosmesis. In addition, an amputee with a large abdomen may encounter difficulty with the pelvic band. If the abdomen, or "roll" is large enough to fit under the pelvic band while standing, during sitting this soft tissue will get pinched. This is very uncomfortable for the amputee and may be a contraindiction for using this system. For amputees who need the extra lateral support and can tolerate the discomfort of the pinching of the soft tissue on the anterior wall of the socket during sitting, the hip joint and pelvic band is a reliable and effective suspension system.

In addition to the conventional hip joint, which is usually made of steel or aluminum, newer hip joints are made from plastic. The plastic hip joints can only be used if the amputee has a stable hip. The main advantage of the plastic hip joint is weight reduction, but it will not produce the same degree of mediolateral stability as metal.

Suction

No other above-knee prosthetic suspension system gets more notoriety than suction. The suction system is one in which the amputee does not wear a stump sock but has direct and total contact of the skin with the socket. A one-way valve, usually located in the anteromedial corner of the socket, allows air to be expelled from the socket when the stump is inserted, causing a negative pressure within the socket (Fig. 5–13). This pressure, sealed by perspiration, and the friction force of the skin against the socket walls keep the limb in place.

Many amputees start out with another type of suspension and ultimately ask for suction. It is not without problems. The use of suction demands an intimate fit between the residual limb and the socket. This assumes that the volume of the stump is constant and will not change. It is therefore not a suspension system that may be readily used in a temporary device. The use of suction also can be troublesome if there are fluctuations in the amputee's body weight. Often amputees are in a state of either losing weight or trying to lose weight, making the use of suction difficult. Another consideration in the use of suction is the ability of the amputee to don or to put on the limb independently. The process of donning the suction socket requires some skill and good balance. Amputees often use a "pull sock," which is placed on the stump and pulled through the valve opening while the stump is being inserted into the socket. Sometimes the amputee will stand in a corner to make certain that he or she does not fall. Amputees having had recent cataract surgery for whom high pressure caused by the Valsalva maneuver is a problem, are not candidates for suction suspension.

Although the suction socket tends to make the prosthetic limb feel more like part of the amputee, it is not uncommon to use auxiliary suspension to ensure that the limb will not come off, particularly when the amputee is away from home or at work. To this end a Silesian band may be applied just in case the suction breaks. Tight-fitting pants, often worn by younger amputees, can provide another form of auxiliary suspension for the suction socket. A total elastic suspension (TES) belt is also popular.

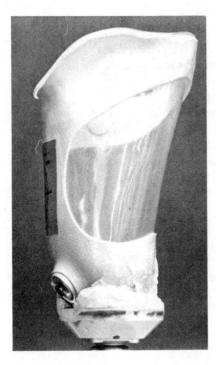

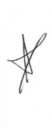

Figure 5–13. A suction above-knee socket.

Since suction suspension tends to work better with compact, muscular, residual limbs, young, active amputees are often effective users of this type of suspension. It is usually preferred by almost all amputees who use it. Suction will, however, produce skin problems, due in part to the high forces that occur between the socket and the skin, particularly in the posteromedial corner. The medial wall may also pinch if the amputee is not careful to pull all the adductor skin into the socket every time the limb is applied. Sebaceous cysts are common in the medial and posterior regions, and once they occur they tend to reoccur. Unfortunately the best treatment for this type of problem is rest outside of the socket, with the amputee not wearing the limb during this period of healing. New amputees who inquire about suction should be told about potential problems to allow them to make an informed decision as to whether the additional benefits are worth the potential pain and discomfort.

MANAGEMENT OF THE RESIDUAL LIMB

As with below-knee amputees, the surgeon determines the postoperative care of the wound. Shaping and conditioning of the stump is accomplished using two principal techniques: rigid dressings and compression wraps.

Rigid Dressings

Rigid dressing for the above-knee stump, as originally described by Burgess,[11] was used in the late 1960s and early 1970s. However, it never gained the overall popularity of the below-knee system due mainly to the difficulty and complexity of suspending the above-knee rigid dressing. The system was identical to the below-knee system, except that the suspension of the cast was accomplished via cables, referred to as Bowden cables, connected to a waist belt. Suspension was less than ideal, and a great deal of effort and patience were required by both the prosthetist and the amputee.

Thorpe et al,[12] in 1979, reported a prospective study on the use of rigid dressings in above-knee amputees. The rigid dressings were applied by either a physical therapist or prosthetist. Results showed that rigid dressings were beneficial no matter who applied them as long as that person was properly trained in the procedure. Additionally, the study reported that early ambulation usually necessitated greater use of pain medication, indicating that early ambulation was not advisable. No problems with wound healing could be attributed to the rigid dressing or to the treatment regimen or person applying the device.

Compression Wrapping

Generally the postoperative routine for above-knee amputees today does not include the use of a rigid dressing. Instead the above-knee amputee is taught to use a compression wrap for four to six weeks (Fig. 5–14). The spica component of the thigh-wrapping procedure is essential for proper suspension of the wrap. Compression of the medial

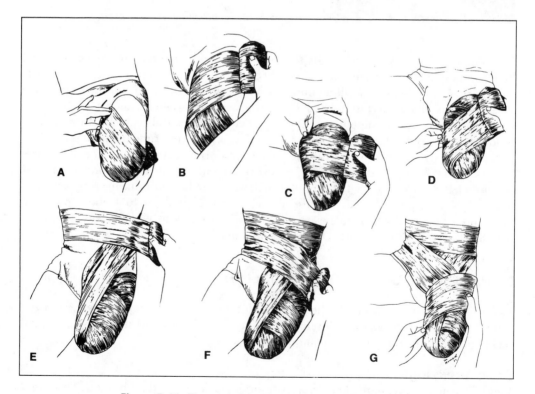

Figure 5–14. Figure-of-eight, above-knee compression wrap.

thigh or adductor region is likewise very important. If wrapping is difficult, a stump shrinker is easily applied.

Following this time the amputee is fitted with a temporary prosthesis that has a quadrilateral socket (Fig. 5–15). Since complete shrinking of the above-knee residual limb may take six to 12 months, the socket allows the amputee to learn to walk with a prosthesis while the residual limb is continuing to shrink. The amputee can continue to add stump socks as the volume changes.

The short and very short above-knee amputation levels usually present many problems. Compression wrapping at this level is virtually impossible, since suspension of the wrap is quite difficult, even using proper techniques. There is simply too little residual limb to either wrap or to grasp. Care must be exercised not to overemphasize the importance of stump wrapping, since the amount of edema usually present at this level is not a major problem.

Other Factors Affecting the Residual Limb

Factors that may affect the residual limb at the above-knee level are similar to those at the below-knee level, as discussed in Chapter 4.

In cases where an above-knee amputation is performed for such reasons as an infected internal fixator or plate, the wound may need to be left open for five to seven

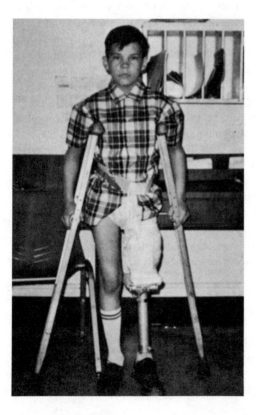

Figure 5–15. Temporary above-knee prosthesis.

days following surgery to allow the wound to clean up and to rid the wound of the infection. Following that period a secondary closure usually is done. This treatment is most successful in young, otherwise healthy people who heal without delay. When these problems coexist with vascular disease or diabetes, the result may not always be as positive.

In some traumatic cases in which there is denuding of the skin over the residual limb, skin grafts may be required. This makes the surgical procedure difficult, since there is a need to maintain as much length as possible and to surgically close the wound as quickly as possible to prevent further chance of infection. In young children there is often considerable effort to preserve growth plates so as not to create a serious leg-length discrepancy. Skin grafting slows down the overall management process and can leave scar tissue that is not very mobile. Tethered or grafted skin without normal mobility makes prosthetic fitting difficult, tending to cause splits or ulcers on the residual limb. Such ulceration should not be misinterpreted as being caused by the prosthesis, when actually the skin simply split due to its need to stretch. Amputees can walk on prostheses while having splits in grafted skin as long as everyone involved knows what caused the split and the wound itself is kept clean until it heals. Skin grafts from trauma or burns may take a long time to finally heal. Careful observation of such cases can allow the amputee to begin using an above-knee prosthesis while not bringing further harm to the residual limb.

A major problem associated with management of the above-knee residual limb is hip-flexion contracture. The more severe the hip flexion contracture the more difficult the prosthetic fitting, and the more difficult acceptance of the prosthesis will be for the amputee. Severe contractures, in excess of 25 degrees, cause unsightly cosmetic problems for the amputee. The prosthetist can accommodate a relatively large hip-flexion contracture by increased preflexing of the socket within the prosthesis, but there are compromises that have to be made. In sitting, when the prosthesis rests on the chair, a markedly preflexed socket produces an anterior bulge under the pants or dress and does not allow for the even accommodation of a tray or other object placed on the amputee's lap.

Excessive hip flexion contractures also cause problems for the use of prosthetic knees. Since most prosthetic knees require weight bearing to stabilize them in stance phase, the "flexed" orientation of the prosthetic knee makes the use of other than "locked" knees difficult. This of course limits which prosthetic knees are available to the amputee, since they have to be locked to produce stability in stance phase. The amputee with a severe hip-flexion contracture may also be required to take a shortened step with the sound limb because of his or her inability to extend the prosthetic limb during the late stance phase of gait.

A common complicating factor affecting the postoperative management of the above-knee amputee is the presence of edema and its associated prosthetic problems. The quadrilateral socket is designed around the concept that the limb may get smaller due to shrinking or edema absorption but not that the limb will get larger due to edema. When the limb swells, fewer stump socks may be worn, but often the socket is not large enough to accommodate the residual limb even with no stump socks. It is not uncommon to see amputees who vary in volume from day to day or hour to hour and who make limb fitting difficult. Included in this group are amputees with arteriovenous malformations; their residual limb changes size hourly and they often need two sockets, one for when the residual limb is swollen and one for after it drains and becomes smaller.

ALIGNMENT OF THE ABOVE-KNEE PROSTHESIS

As with below-knee prostheses, alignment of an above-knee prosthesis refers to the positioning or state of adjustment of the prosthetic parts in relation to each other and occurs in two phases: static, or bench, and dynamic. With below-knee alignment, the focus is primarily on the relationship between the socket and the prosthetic foot. With above-knee alignment the presence of a prosthetic knee joint poses some additional considerations. Also in the above-knee prosthesis, attention must be paid to the influences that prosthetic alignment may have on the hip, since this joint is important to proper functioning of the prosthesis.

Stability of the Prosthetic Knee

An important reference used in the alignment of above-knee prostheses is a vertical (plumb) line originating from the greater trochanter of the residual limb. Since in the lateral view this line passes very close to the prosthetic knee axis and the (hypothetical) ankle axis, it is generally referred to as the trochanter-knee-ankle line or, more simply, the TKA line (Fig. 5–16). The relative position of the TKA line, either in front or back of the knee-joint center, determines the relative stability of the knee in the stance phase of gait. If this line falls in front of the knee center, the knee is described as stable, meaning that there is a net gravitational extension moment when weight is placed on the prosthesis in an upright position. This situation, sometimes referred to as negative TKA alignment, demands a greater hip flexion moment to initiate prosthetic knee flexion during swing phase. If the TKA line falls behind the knee joint center, the knee will tend to buckle from the gravitational moment applied to it as the amputee bears weight on the limb. This assumes that the knee is free to flex and that the amputee is exerting no hip extension moment to the prosthesis to nullify the gravitational knee-flexion moment. The condition in which the prosthetic knee-joint-center is exactly on the TKA line is referred to as a "trigger" condition, meaning that the knee is in stable but easily perturbed alignment.

Prosthetic knee components are inherently stable in extension, with mechanical stops or locking mechanisms preventing, or at least limiting, hyperextension. If the prosthetic knee is working properly, there is no medial or lateral motion.

Mediolateral Stability of the Hip

In addition to knee stability, hip stability is an important concern for the above-knee amputee. In the quadrilateral socket the ischial tuberosity is the main point of weight bearing and may be thought of as a pivot on the top of the posterior wall. During single-limb support on the prosthetic side, the body weight, located medially to the pivot point, causes an adduction moment of the pelvis on the femur. To neutralize this moment an equal and opposite moment produced by the hip abductors is necessary to

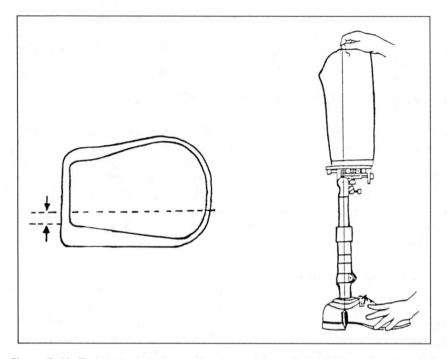

Figure 5–16. The trochanter-knee-ankle reference line. (From Northwestern University Prosthetic Orthotic Center, 1987, with permission.)

maintain the pelvis level. If the amputee is unable or unwilling, because of discomfort, to generate an adequate hip moment, he or she may lean or list in the direction of the prosthesis to minimize the adduction moment and, consequently, the hip abductor force needed to counteract it. By preadducting the femur to approximately 7 degrees, the hip abductors are placed in a position of stretch, affording some advantage. The length of the above-knee stump determines how large an area is available for distribution of the hip abductor force. In the event that the area is too small or that the force produced is inadequate, a hip joint and pelvic-band suspension may be added to augment mediolateral hip stability during stance phase.

Above-Knee Bench Alignment

Bench alignment of the above-knee prosthesis provides a place to start. It represents the prosthetist's best guess at initial alignment and generally satisfies most amputee's early gait requirements. Changes usually need to be made as training progresses. Classic bench alignment for a medium-length residual limb must be considered from both the posterior and lateral views (Fig. 5–17). Posteriorly the center of the heel falls just under the point of ischial seat contact. Laterally the knee center will be on "trigger," with the lateral TKA line passing through the knee center and the ankle center. The knee bolt should be 5 degrees externally rotated from the line of progression and horizontal. This will allow the shank portion of the prosthesis to swing straight forward and prevent knee whips.

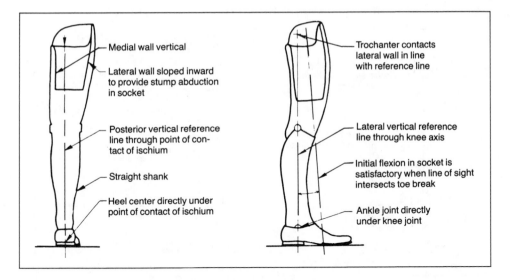

Figure 5–17. Lateral and posterior alignment for medium functional length above-knee residual limb. (From Radcliffe CW. Functional considerations in the fitting of above-knee prostheses. *Art Limbs*. 1955; **2**:40, with permission.)

Figure 5–18 shows that the socket is generally abducted in the case of a short residual limb. This is done to provide a wider, safer base of support, since the amputee is likely to have more difficulty controlling the prosthesis with the short stump. The center of the heel is outset relative to a perpendicular line from the ischial tuberosity to the floor. Laterally the knee center will be aligned posteriorly of the TKA line, making the knee more stable.

Figure 5–19 shows that with a long above-knee stump the shank and foot are inset relative to a reference line from the ischial tuberosity to the floor. This, in effect, narrows the base of support. The longer length of the femur allows for enough abduction force to balance the pelvis in stance phase. Laterally, although the amount of preflexion of the socket is limited by the length of the residual limb, the ankle joint is aligned behind the knee joint, with the lateral TKA falling through or just behind the knee center, allowing marginal stability but easy initiation of swing phase.

Above-Knee Dynamic Alignment

Gait characteristics may be altered using an adjustable alignment device. If any such alteration proves to be difficult or undesirable, a return to the original alignment is easily accomplished.

FUNCTIONAL TRAINING OF THE ABOVE-KNEE AMPUTEE

Functional training of the above-knee amputee is not unlike training of the below-knee amputee. However, in the case of the above-knee amputee, the hip joint significantly affects how the amputee is likely to function using a prosthesis. For this reason a

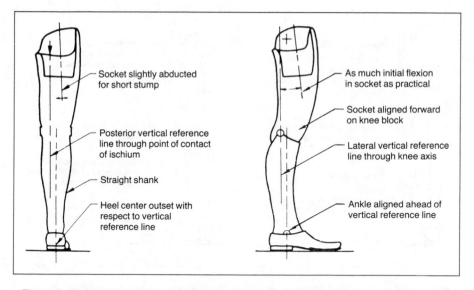

Figure 5–18. Lateral and posterior alignment for short functional length above-knee residual limb. (From Radcliffe CW. Functional considerations in the fitting of above-knee prostheses. *Art Limbs.* 1955; **2**:40, with permission.)

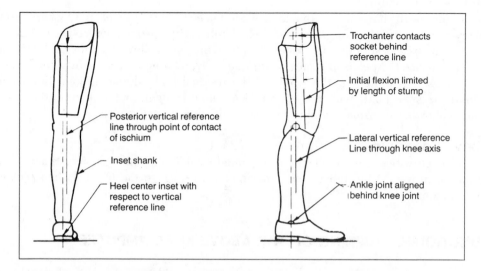

Figure 5–19. Lateral and posterior alignment for long functional length above-knee residual limb. (From Radcliffe CW. Functional considerations in the fitting of above-knee prostheses. *Art Limbs.* 1955; **2**:40, with permission.)

thorough evaluation of the hip should be done and as much remedial work as possible should be begun prior to fitting the definitive limb. It is, however, permissible to proceed with the fitting of the temporary device, as it often contributes to the resolution of some problems, such as a hip flexion contracture, by forcing the hip to stretch during each step in gait.

During the early preprosthetic days following the above-knee amputation, care should be taken to prevent any tightness or contracture in the hip joint, as contractures are more easily prevented than treated. The test for tightness of the hip, the Thomas test, tests for both the presence of hip flexion contracture and the amount of hip joint range of motion. With the amputee supine with pelvis square, a hand is placed under the lumbar spine while flexing the residual limb up toward the trunk. As the hip flexes, the point where the back flattens is the limit of hip flexion. Full hip flexion is 135 degrees and allows the limb to touch the abdomen. With the sound leg resting against the abdomen, any inability of the amputee to flatten the residual limb to the examination table without reinitiation of the lumbar lordosis may indicate the presence of a hip flexion contracture. Experience has taught that many geriatric amputees, particularly above-knee amputees, do not cooperate with the test, since it is physically difficult to do so. It is also necessary to recommend prone lying to stretch the hip flexors and to prevent or retard any hip-flexor tightness.

In addition to evaluating hip flexors and extensors, the hip abductors are also an important muscle group. The hip abductors play a key role in the amputee's ability to stabilize the pelvis in stance phase of gait. Without the hip abductors, the amputee will lean to the amputated side and produce a cosmetically unacceptable gait as well as expend greater energy. It is important to remember when testing the hip abductors that both hips should remain in a neutral position, since any hip flexion allows the hip flexors to substitute for the abductors and gives the examiner an erroneous impression of the strength of the abductors. Sidelying is another way of testing the strength of the abductors, maintaining the hip in neutral, with the amputated side up.

When using SA, constant-friction exoskeletal prosthetic components, the stability of the knee in stance phase is directly related to the amputee's ability to generate a hip extension moment at the initiation of heel strike, to maintain the pelvis in a neutral position, and also to generate a force larger than the force tending to flex the knee. It is important the patient be taught very early in gait training about the need for the extension force generated by the residual limb at the hip to prevent the knee from buckling. As was described in regard to alignment, the more posteriorly placed the knee center, the more inherent stability there is in the prosthesis. Conversely, greater stability also makes the initiation of knee flexion in swing phase more difficult.

Just as with the below-knee amputee, it is important during the early period of functional training that the amputee learns about the proper fit of the socket, what the proper fit feels like, and how to modify the fit to make it more comfortable.

KNEE DISARTICULATION

The major disadvantage of the knee disarticulation prosthesis is the outside knee hinges, since the end of the femur occupies the space in the prosthesis usually occupied by the prosthetic knee unit. It is imperative that the amputee not have a pre-existing hip flexion contracture, since the prosthetic limb will be quite long. Figure 5–20 shows the outside hinges on the knee of the prosthesis. One can also understand that the alignment of such a device demands that the leg be adducted so the base is not excessively wide.

If outside hinges are not used, a four-bar linkage knee may be considered. As seen in Figure 5–21, the design of the four-bar–linkage knee unit places the knee center of rotation as close to the end of the residual limb as possible. Thus as the prosthetic knee flexes, the changing center of the knee approximates the end of the socket. This produces a very cosmetically acceptable knee length, visable when the amputee is sitting with the thighs together. If it were not for this four-bar linkage, the knee centers would not be even in sitting, with the knee disarticulation prosthesis extending out beyond the sound side knee.

The socket designed for the through-knee amputation accepts most of the weight bearing on the end of the residual limb. In swing phase of gait, suspension of the device comes from the molding of the socket over the femoral condyles. If the distal end of the residual limb is bulbous, a trap door-type socket may be used. This socket design is very similar to that used for the Syme's amputation and for the very same reason. Once the amputee dons the socket, the door is closed over the femoral condyles, thus suspending the prosthesis.

Baumgartner[13] believes that the knee disarticulation should be considered in every patient for whom short below-knee amputation is not possible, in spite of the age or

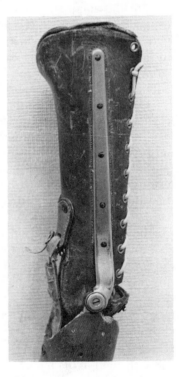

Figure 5–20. A lateral view of a leather knee-disarticulation prosthesis with outside knee hinges.

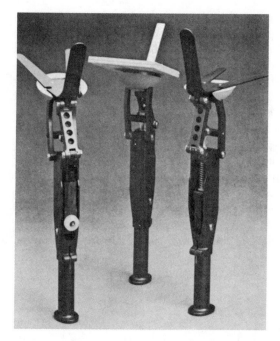

Figure 5–21. Lyquist's Orthopaedic Hospital of Copenhagen (OHC) four-bar linkage knee.

etiology of the patient. He prefers to leave the entire femur and the patella and recommends that the gastrocnemius be completely removed.

Prosthetic gait problems of the knee disarticulation level include knee stability in early stance phase and the initiation of knee flexion in late stance phase. Greene[6] compares several commercially available four-bar linkage knees, contrasting them as to design stability.

ENERGY EXPENDITURE AND GAIT IN ABOVE-KNEE AMPUTEES

As is true with the literature on below-knee amputees, there are no studies of energy expenditure during gait in above-knee amputees, which separate the contributions of vascular disease from the effects of having an above-knee amputation and prosthesis. Waters[14] studied 13 vascular and 15 traumatic above-knee amputees and found that the vascular amputees walked 36 m/min, or 65% of normal speed. The dysvascular above-knee amputees used 12.6 mL O_2/kg·min to walk 36m/min. The 12.6 mL O_2/kg·min is approximately equal to the normal predicted rate as described by Corcoran[15]; however, the walking speed is greatly reduced, from 80 m/min to 36 m/min. Traumatic above-knee amputees fared better using 12.9 mL O_2 kg·min while walking at a rate of 52 m/min. The O_2 use is up a bit from the 12.65 normal value at 80 m/min. The traumatic above-knee amputees walked 52 m/min or 45% of normal.

James,[16] in his study of 37 above-knee amputees aged 21 to 62 years, none of whom were vascular in origin, found that they walked 30% slower than normal, using 61 kcal/

kg·min. In a recent article by Otis et al,[17] energy cost during gait was compared between osteosarcoma victims with resection and prosthetic replacement and amputation above the knee. Results indicate that the patient with resection/prosthetic replacement had lower energy costs during gait. Detailed data concerning the components of the above-knee limbs, however, were not presented. Specifically, free walking speed of resection/replacement patients was 87% (54 m/min) of normal, with the above-knee amputees at 73% (45 m/min), with normal measured at 62 m/min. However, 62 m/min is 22% less than accepted, normal walking speed. At free-speed walking, the relative energy costs were 160% of normal for the resection/replacement group and 209% for the amputees. Compared with Waters[14] this study resulted in a larger net-energy cost for the above-knee amputees (0.30 +/− 0.05 mL/kg·m to 0.25 +/− 0.05 mL/kg·m). Other results of gait speed, reported by Fisher,[18] vary from 20% slower to 66% slower, from 70 m/min to 28.2 m/min. The associated increase in energy expenditure ranged from 30% to 120% of normal. As is true of below-knee amputees, above-knee amputees, even under the best of circumstances, must expand a great deal of additional energy during ambulation.

REFERENCES

1. Aitken GT. *Courses on Juvenile Prosthetics.* Northwestern University Medical School, 1974.
2. Kay HW, Newman JD. Relative incidences of new amputations. *Orthot Prosthet.* 1975; **29**(2):3–16.
3. McCollough NC, Jennings JJ, Sarmiento A. Bilateral below the knee amputations in patients over fifty years of age. *J Bone Joint Surg.* 1972; **54A**(6):1217–1223.
4. Shea JD. Surgical techniques for lower extremity amputation. *Orthop Clin North Am.* 1972; 3(2):287–301.
5. Mooney V. Above knee amputation, surgical procedures. In: *Atlas of Limb Prosthetics.* St. Louis, MO: Mosby; 1981: 378–401.
6. Greene MP. Four-bar linkage knee analysis. *Orthot Prosthet.* 1983; **37**:(1)15–24.
7. Lehneis HR. Prosthetic Update: 1980 *Newsletter: Prosthet and Orthot Clinic.* 1980; 4(1):1–2.
8. Radcliffe CW. Above-knee prosthetics. *Prosthet Orthot Int.* 1977; 1(1):146–160.
9. Breakey JW. Flexible below knee socket with supracondylar suspension. *Orthot Prosthet.* 1970; **24**(1):1–10.
10. Kristinsson O. Flexible above knee socket made from low density polyethylene suspended by a weight transmitting frame. *Orthot Prosthet.* 1983; **37**(2):25–27.
11. Burgess EM, Romano RL, Zettl JH, Schrock RD. Amputations of the leg for peripheral vascular insufficiency. *J Bone Joint Surg.* 1971; **53A**(5):874–890.
12. Thorpe W, et al: A prospective study of the rehabilitation of the above knee amputee with rigid dressings. *Clin Orthop.* 1979; **143**:133–137.
13. Baumgartner RF. Knee disarticulation versus above-knee amputation. *Prosthet Orthot Int.* 1984; 3(1):15–19.
14. Waters RL, Perry J, Antonelli D, Hislop H. Energy cost of walking of amputees: Influence of level of amputation. *J Bone Joint Surg.* 1976; **58A**:42–46.
15. Corcoran PJ, Brengelmann GL. Oxygen uptake in normal and handicapped subjects in relation to speed of walking beside velocity controlled cart. *Arch Phys Med Rehab.* 1970; **51**:78–87.

16. James U. Oxygen uptake and heart rate during prosthetic walking in healthy male unilateral above-knee amputees. *Scand J Rehabil Med.* 1973; **5**:71–80.

17. Otis JC, Lane JM, Kroll MA: Energy cost during gait in osteosarcoma patients after resection and knee replacement and after above-the-knee amputation. *J Bone Joint Surg.* 1985; **67A**(4):606–611.

18. Fisher SV, Gullickson G. Energy cost of ambulation in health and disability: A literature review. *Arch Phys Med Rehabil.* 1978; **59**:124–133.

CHAPTER 6

Hip Disarticulation Amputation

This chapter discusses hip disarticulation amputations. This type of amputation is not commonly encountered in a typical general hospital setting. However, when it is seen, it represents unique challenges that are distinct from the routine management of other amputees. This chapter is intended as an overview of factors to be kept in mind when dealing with these special situations.

HIP DISARTICULATION/HEMIPELVECTOMY AMPUTATIONS

Most authors and surgeons agree that any thigh amputation of less than 5 cm in length constitutes a functional hip disarticulation. It is important to keep in mind the distinction between an anatomic level and a prosthetic level. The very short above-knee anatomic level cannot function as an above-knee prosthetic level. Functionally, therefore, it can be considered as a hip disarticulation prosthetic level.

Etiology

Hip disarticulation and hemipelvectomy represent radical forms of surgery that are rarely performed and only when other treatment alternatives are not available. Many authors give the impression that such radical surgery is always done secondary to a malignancy. For example, the 1975 revised edition of New York University's Limb Prosthetic Manual states that radical procedures such as hip disarticulation and hemipelvectomy are performed "in the rare instances in which amputation is required by trauma or nonmalignant disease."[1] The results of a study by Shurr et al[2] indicated that the most common cause of amputation at the hip disarticulation level was tumor (48%). Other etiologies include infection (20%), vascular disease (20%), trauma (10%), and congenital abnormalities (2%; Table 6–1). These data support the contention that hip disarticulations are performed for many of the same reasons as other lower-extremity amputations.

Table 6–2 cites the literature reporting the results of prosthetic fittings of patients with hemipelvectomies done because of tumor. User percentages vary from 6% to 80% in groups ranging in size from 10 to 60 patients. In most cases the primary focus of the reports was not prosthetic, and therefore the data were not well developed.

TABLE 6-1. INDICATIONS FOR HIP DISARTICULATION OR HEMIPELVECTOMY

Indications	Number of Patients (%)	Number Fitted	Number of Users at Follow-up
Tumor	24 (48%)	9	8*
Infection	10 (20%)	1	0
Trauma	5 (10%)	4	3
Congenital	1 (2%)	1	1
Vascular	10 (20%)	0	0
Total	50	15	12

*Three died following fitting, although prosthetic use was documented prior to death.
From Shurr, DG et al. Hip disarticulation. A prosthetic follow-up. Orthot Prosthet. *1984;37:52.*

In a report by Sneppen et al[8] on consecutive cases done for malignant tumors, hip-disarticulation prosthetic fitting occurred in 30 of the 41 patients. Six patients were primarily supplied with prostheses using leather bucket-type sockets (Fig. 6–1) and 24 with Canadian style hip-disarticulation (CHD) prostheses (Fig. 6–2).

There has been some discussion about the philosophical problems faced by surgeons regarding the prosthetic fitting of children having amputations done for tumors. In 1972 Lambert[9] studied a group of 85 children with primary bone tumors, and concluded that since the average wear time was 15.5 months per case, the cost of prosthetic fitting was justified in all cases. Unfortunately he made no record of whether the children began with a prosthesis and then discontinued use prior to death or surgery or were alive and well and not using a prosthesis at follow-up. This group included 11 upper-limb prostheses; Lambert's study does not deal with any problems encountered in lower-limb prosthetic fitting or wearing at follow-up.

Hip Disarticulation/Hemipelvectomy Prostheses

The most commonly used hip disarticulation prosthesis is the CHD version, introduced by McClaurin[10] in 1957. More recently the Otto Bock modular (OBM) endoskeletal version has been employed because of lighter overall weight, improved cosmesis, and the opportunity to use interchangeable and adjustable components (Fig. 6–3).

TABLE 6-2. PERCENTAGE OF FITTED PATIENTS USING HIP DISARTICULATION PROSTHESES

Author(s)	Date	Number of Patients Fitted	Number of Patients Using at F/U
Lewis and Bickel[3]	1957	25	2 (8%)
Miller[4]	1959	32	22 (69%)
Watkins[5]	1962	10	8 (80%)
Higinbothom et al[6]	1966	60	24 (40%)
Douglas et al[7]	1975	50	3 (6%)
Sneppen et al[8]	1978	30	15 (50%)
Shurr et al[2]	1983	15	12 (80%)

From Shurr, DG et al. Hip disarticulation. A prosthetic follow-up. Orthot Prosthet. *1984;37:52.*

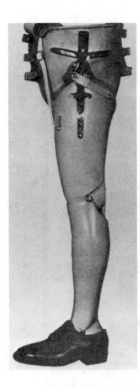

Figure 6–1. Hip disarticulation prosthesis with leather bucket-type socket. (From *Orthopaedic Appliances Atlas, Artifical Limbs.* Ann Arbor, MI: JW Edwards, 1960;2, with permission.)

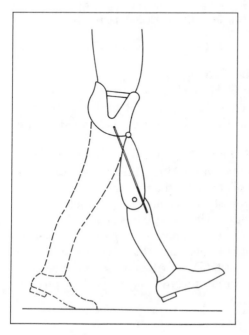

Figure 6–2. CHD prosthesis. (From Northwestern University Prosthetic Orthotic Center, 1987, with permission.)

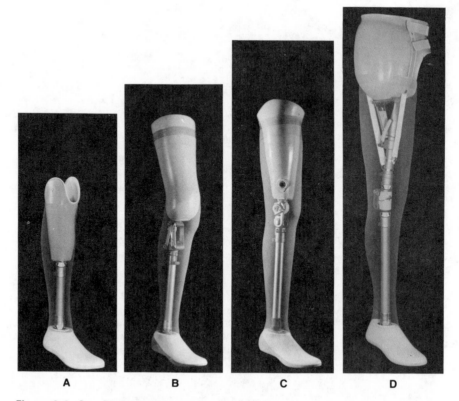

Figure 6–3. Otto Bock modular lower extremity prosthesis: **(A)** below knee; **(B)** knee disarticulation; **(C)** above knee; **(D)** hip disarticulation. (From Otto Bock Orthopedic Industry, Inc., Minneapolis, MN, with permission.)

Etiological Factors Affecting Prosthetic Fitting

Criteria for hip disarticulation-level prosthetic fitting include a patient who (1) has a healed wound; (2) can expend the energy needed for ambulation; (3) desires to learn to walk with a prosthesis; and (4) has no illness at the time of fitting that would negate learning how to use a prosthesis.

In a study by Shurr et al[2] (Table 6–2), 15 of 60 (25%) patients were fitted with a prosthesis. Most of these patients had an amputation for either tumor (nine cases) or trauma (four cases). In only one of the 10 cases of amputation done for infection did the patient's overall medical condition allow for a realistic expectation of prosthetic fitting. One congenital hip-disarticulation patient was fitted with a prosthesis at age 16 months, without difficulty. None of the 10 patients who had an amputation for vascular reasons was fitted with a prosthesis. One trauma patient was not fitted because of severe depression. Patients who had demonstrable metastatic chest lesions were not considered to be prosthetic candidates. For this last group the time of death after surgery ranged from three to 60 months.

Incidence of Prosthetic Use

In the study by Shurr et al,[2] the initial time of the four patients with trauma-induced amputations ranged from one to three months after injury. Three learned to use the prosthesis readily and continued to use it at follow-up, ranging from 15 to 24 months. The fourth patient also had a shoulder disarticulation and an above-knee amputation on the other lower extremity. His gait training was understandably difficult, and at follow-up he reported that the energy costs were too great for the benefit derived.

The one fitted patient whose amputation had been caused by infection discontinued wear of his prosthesis after two months because of discomfort in the socket and around the waist. All nine of the fitted patients, whose cause of amputation was tumor, learned to use the prosthesis without difficulty. Three of these patients died secondary to their disease. Time of prosthesis use prior to death ranged from 11 to 60 months. The remaining six patients were alive and well at follow-up, with five of them still using a prosthetic device.

Other Factors Affecting Prosthetic Use

In addition to etiology and level of amputation, some authors have alluded to a possible decreasing interest in prosthetic usage associated with age. To date, no research has clearly documented this trend, if it exists.

Assuming a suitable candidate, the success of prosthetic use is likely to also depend upon (1) prosthetic socket fit; (2) the patient's ability to walk independently enough to free his or her hands from assistive devices; (3) the limited need for sitting with the prosthesis for long periods; and (4) the lack of relative changes in body weight and size.

Questions concerning the different types of hip-disarticulation prostheses and the subjective evaluation of these devices have only been preliminarily addressed by Shurr et al.[2] Of four patients fitted with CHD prostheses, two were subsequently fitted with the OBM system. Both patients' responses were positive and based mainly on the improved cosmesis and soft cover. The apparent lighter weight was also a positive factor. Likewise, the location of the hip joint and uncomfortable sitting were sources of concern. Otto Bock has recently developed the 7E7 hip joint, which addresses this problem.

Training of the Hip Disarticulation Amputee

Only the article by Watkins[5] discusses the number of visits necessary to teach a hip-disarticulation amputee to walk at an acceptable level. His comparisons were between leather "tilt-table" sockets, the then-new CHD prosthesis, and the OBM prosthesis. An average of 20 visits for physical therapy were necessary to achieve independent gait with the tilt-table socket. An average of 17 visits were necessary to achieve independent gait with the CHD, with or without a cane. An average of nine sessions were required to achieve independent use of the OBM, with or without a cane.

Gait using crutches should be a less-than-acceptable outcome for gait training because the prosthesis normally can be used without requiring upper-extremity assistance. The inability to use the upper limbs may often be a contributing factor in prosthesis rejection.

Improvements in the biomechanics of hip disarticulation prostheses have made learning to walk easier and faster. More research is needed to better define this patient group and to identify further prosthetic and ambulatory problems experienced with long-term use of hip disarticulation prostheses.

REFERENCES

1. Lower-limb prosthetics. New York: New York University Medical School; 1975:243.
2. Shurr DG, Cook TM, Buckwalter JA, Cooper RR. Hip disarticulation: A prosthetic follow-up. *Orthot Prosthet.* 1984; **37**(1):50–57.
3. Lewis R, Bickel W. Hemipelvectomy for malignant disease. *J Am Med Assoc.* 1957; **165**:8–12.
4. Miller T. Interiho-abdominal amputation. A report of 32 cases. *Acta Radiol (Stockh).* 1959; **188** (Suppl):173–189.
5. Watkins A. Rehabilitation after hemipelvectomy. *J Am Med Assoc.* 1962; **181**:793–794.
6. Higinbotham N, Marcove R, Casson P. Hemipelvectomy: A clinical study of 100 cases with five years follow-up on 60 patients. *Surgery.* 1971; **59**:706–708.
7. Douglas H, Razack M, Holyoke E. Hemipelvectomy. *Arch Surg.* 1975; **110**:82–85.
8. Sneppen O, Johansen T, Heerfordt J, Dissing I, Peterson O. Hemipelvectomy. *Acta Orthop Scand.* 1978; **49**:175–179.
9. Lambert CT. Amputation surgery in the child. *Ortho Clin North Am.* 1972; 3(2):476.
10. McLaurin CA. The evolution of the Canadian-type hip disarticulation prosthesis. *Art Limb.* 1957; 4:22–28.

CHAPTER 7

Lower Limb Orthotics

This chapter begins with a discussion of the users of and functions provided by lower limb orthotic devices. It then presents various orthotic configurations, beginning with foot orthotics and ending with hip-knee-ankle-foot orthoses. A brief consideration of fracture orthoses is also included. This chapter assumes that the reader is thoroughly familiar with the terms and concepts found in Chapters 1, 2, and 3. In particular, the reader should be familiar with the universal terminology for describing orthotic devices (Chapter 1); with the methods, materials, and general mechanical considerations common to most orthotic applications (Chapter 2); and with the functional tasks that comprise normal human gait (Chapter 3).

USERS OF LOWER LIMB ORTHOTICS

A wide variety of physical impairments can result in lower limb dysfunction. Table 7–1 lists some of the major impairments that may result in an individual who could benefit from the application of a lower limb orthosis.

FUNCTIONS OF A LOWER LIMB ORTHOSIS

Lower limb orthoses can provide one or more of the following functions:

1. Maintenance or correction of body segment *alignment*.
2. Assistance or resistance to joint *motion*.
3. Axial loading and therefore relief of *weight bearing*.
4. *Protection* against physical insult. 1°athletes & arthritics

It is important for the clinic team to approach each new case without preconceived ideas about the type of device to be prescribed. An accurate and complete assessment must be done to determine the patient's existing functional abilities and to define precisely the functions to be provided by the orthosis.[1] Use of a standardized form can aid in obtaining all of the necessary information. Development of a successful prescrip-

TABLE 7-1. MAJOR IMPAIRMENTS REQUIRING LOWER LIMB ORTHOTICS

Problems at Birth	Diseases	Trauma
Cerebral palsy	Stroke	Spinal cord injury
Spina bifida	Muscular dystrophy	Fracture
Long bone malformations	Arthritis	Head injuries
Hemophilia	Multiple sclerosis	Muscle, cartilage, and tendon rupture
Osteogenesis imperfecta	Legg-Calvé-Perthes	
Club foot	Poliomyelitis	

Adapted from Lower Limb Orthotics, A Manual. *Philadelphia, Pa: Rehabilitation Engineering Center, 1978.*

tion depends on a clear understanding of the underlying causes of why a patient functions the way he or she does. The relationship between the patient's performance and physical findings should be clear. A distinction also needs to be made between those "deviations" from normal function that represent a primary loss and those that are volitional and compensatory.[2] As with all orthotic and prosthetic applications, the challenge for the clinic team is to provide the greatest augmentation to a decreased function with the least possible interference to other intact functions and with reasonable cosmesis. Usually some compromises must be made.

FOOT ORTHOSES

In the most general sense, any shoe can be considered to be a foot orthosis (FO). It is an external device applied to the body for the purpose of controlling (or at least distributing) forces and for improving function. Poorly designed and poorly constructed footwear can negatively affect normal function. The same is certainly true when a pathologic condition is present. From the point of view of preventing or ameliorating disabilities, a wide spectrum of possibilities exists for providing special shoes or special shoe modifications.

Diabetes, arthritis, and structural malformations and deficiencies of the foot are the leading problems that require foot orthotics as an integral part of treatment. The next largest category of foot orthotic wearers is probably athletes, and the reader is referred to a review by Glancy[3] regarding the prescription and use of foot orthotics to prevent and to manage foot problems in runners.

ANKLE-FOOT ORTHOTICS

The basic functions of the foot-ankle, as discussed in Chapter 3, are surface adaption, shock absorption, control of the center-of-gravity movement, knee stability, and swing-phase shortening. The purpose for prescribing and applying an ankle-foot orthosis (AFO) usually relates to one or more of these functional tasks.

Shoe-Clasp AFO

The shoe-clasp AFO was developed by the Veterans Administration and consists of a posterior fiberglass upright that is loosely attached to a calf band on one end and to a slotted clasp on the other end that slides over the rearmost portion of the top of the shoe, referred to as the counter of the shoe. Figure 7–1 shows the shoe-clasp AFO. This device is useful for a flaccid drop foot during swing phase that is not affected by heel-cord tightness or spasticity.[4] A sturdy shoe must be used, or the counter of the shoe will break down in a relatively short time. This device is one of the few AFOs that allows surface adaption through inversion and eversion at the subtalar joint, assuming there is some control of these structures.

Single and Double Upright AFOs

Figure 7–2 shows examples of what are often referred to as conventional AFOs, namely, those having one or two metal uprights, usually containing an orthotic "ankle" joint, attached to a specially modified shoe and calf band. There are a variety of ways that the uprights might be attached to the shoe (Fig. 7–3). A standard stirrup is a U-shaped steel plate secured between the heel and sole of the shoe, containing part of the orthotic ankle joint at the top of the "U." A "split" stirrup allows each side to be detached from the shoe portion, providing advantages for donning, doffing, and interchanging shoes. A similar arrangement can be provided by using round, metal uprights, referred to as "calipers," that insert, much like the split stirrup, into holes in the side of the shoe plate. These pivot points then act as the orthotic "ankle" joints but may be a problem because of the incongruency between the anatomic and orthotic joint axes of rotation, as

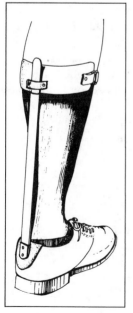

Figure 7–1. VA shoe-clasp AFO.

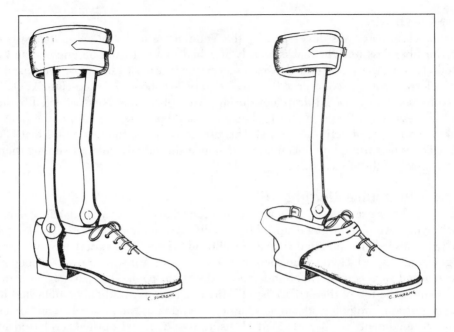

Figure 7–2. Dual-upright and single-upright "conventional" orthoses. Single-upright orthosis also has a "T-strap" for additional mediolateral control of the ankle.

mentioned in Chapter 2. If more stability or control of the foot is required, such as in severe paralysis, a stirrup may contain a metal "sole plate" that extends forward to the metatarsal area (or beyond). Whether the conventional AFO includes single or dual uprights depends on the amount and type of control needed to enhance function. Clearly the dual upright configuration will provide greater medio-lateral stabilization than the single upright othosis.

The "conventional" (double-adjustable or dual-channel) orthotic ankle joint (Fig. 7–4) allows for a number of possibilities, including free motion, a fixed or adjustable dorsiflexion and/or plantarflexion stop using pins, or a dorsiflexion and/or plantarflexion spring assist. Although it is often used as a definitive orthosis, a single or dual upright orthosis provides distinct advantages in terms of adjustability.[5] If an individual's condi-

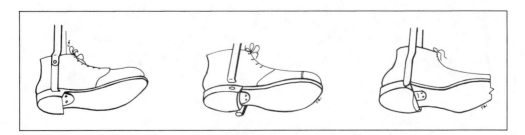

Figure 7–3. Shoe attachments for conventional AFOs.

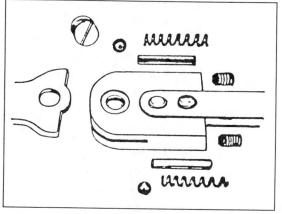

Figure 7–4. Double-adjustable ankle joint.

tion changes due to recovery or deterioration, easy modifications can be made to the device to match changes in the patient's condition. As discussed in Chapter 3, if a specific attitude of the ankle must be chosen, the choice is often a compromise between toe clearance during swing and knee stability during stance. Maintaining a plantarflexed ankle will stabilize the knee during stance but will make the limb longer for swing-phase clearance, while dorsiflexing the ankle will make toe clearance easier but will reduce the stabilizing knee-extension moment during stance phase. The ankle angle will also affect the vertical movement of the center of gravity, although this factor becomes less critical as walking speed is reduced. Structural support of the ankle is not commonly a problem, assuming a reasonable boney alignment can be maintained. If medio-lateral stability of the ankle joint is a problem using a single or dual metal-upright AFO, a "t-strap," as seen in Figure 7–2, can be added to keep the ankle structures in better alignment.

Molded-Shoe Insert AFO

The molded-shoe insert AFO is similar in concept to the conventional single or dual metal-upright AFO except that instead of attaching the orthosis to the shoe by way of a metal stirrup, the lower end of the uprights(s) is attached to a custom-molded plastic-shoe insert (Fig. 7–5). This design allows for all of the same ankle-control possibilities as when using conventional AFOs with the additional advantage that it can provide better valgus or varus control of the foot.[6] It also permits some interchangeability of shoes.

Molded Ankle-Foot Orthosis

Molded ankle-foot orthoses (MAFO) are usually made by vacuum-forming thermoplastic materials, such as polypropylene or polyethylene, over a positive plaster model of the limb. There are a number of design variations that have been used and promulgated by various institutions and individuals. Figure 7–6 shows several examples of different MAFO configurations.

These devices often weigh approximately 150 to 200 g, depending on the size of the individual and the exact design of the device. Usually all portions of the orthosis are in total contact with the shank and foot, providing the possibility for very precise control of

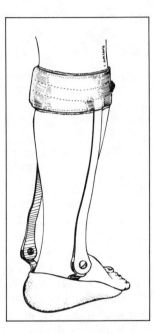

Figure 7–5. Molded shoe-insert AFO.

the limb segments. There are several key variables that are under the control of the orthotist that affect the function of the device, namely, the trimlines of the orthosis, the type of material, the thickness of the material used, and the inclusion of inserts to affect the stiffness at selected locations.

The term "trimline" refers to the various edges where the orthotist cuts or trims the plastic when fabricating the device (Fig. 7–7). If, for instance, the ankle trimline is

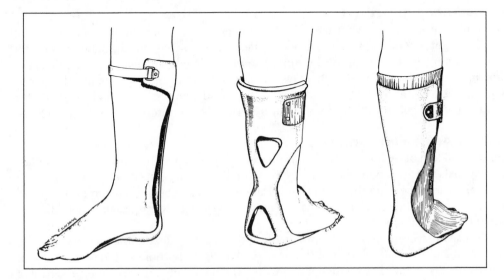

Figure 7–6. Some examples of MAFOs.

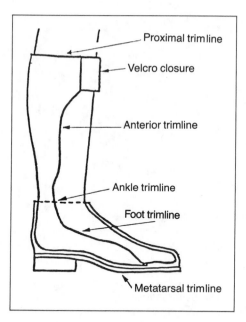

Proximal trimline

Velcro closure

Anterior trimline

Ankle trimline

Foot trimline

Metatarsal trimline

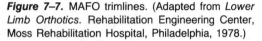

Figure 7–7. MAFO trimlines. (Adapted from *Lower Limb Orthotics.* Rehabilitation Engineering Center, Moss Rehabilitation Hospital, Philadelphia, 1978.)

located anterior to the malleolus, the orthosis will be quite rigid, and only very limited dorsiflexion and plantarflexion will be possible. On the other hand, as more material is trimmed away at the level of the ankle, the orthosis becomes more flexible, allowing more (leaf spring) ankle motion. It is also possible to selectively strengthen or stiffen portions of a plastic orthosis by adding reinforcements of metal, carbon composite, additional sections of polypropylene, or other materials.[7] MAFOs are usually made of polypropylene, but other similar thermoplastic materials such as Lexan (polycarbonate) have been used successfully, and new materials are continually being evaluated as they become available.

Besides the trimlines and the type of material used, the thickness of the sheet of material used during vacuum forming also affects the flexibility and therefore the function of the finished orthosis. Starting thicknesses of from ⅛ to 3/16 in are not uncommon.

The major advantages to a totally plastic MAFO are improved cosmesis, interchangeability of shoes, and extreme lightness. Although some adjustment and reshaping of MAFOs is possible, these devices are not indicated for patients with changing conditions, especially patients with volumetric changes in the limb. Because of the intimate fit of these devices, care should be taken with patients who have decreased sensation, since pressure sores can easily develop. Additionally, severe spasticity with equinus or varus deformity may be a contraindication for use of an MAFO.[4]

In addition to the possible adaptation of standard, conventional ankle joints to MAFOs, several new ankle (and knee) joints have been developed specifically for incorporation into thermoplastic orthoses. Figure 7–8 shows some examples of such joints. Reported advantages using these components include better alignment of the orthotic ankle axis with the anatomic ankle axis, minimal resistance over a selected

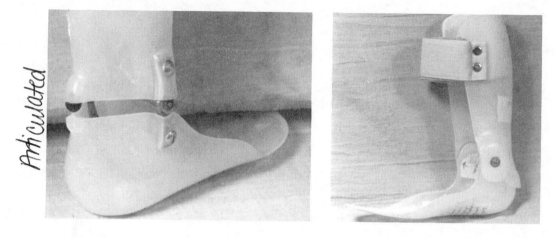

Articulated

Figure 7–8. Examples of ankle joints for MAFOs.

range of motion, and the option for positive, precise stopping action within given limits. Continued development and use of this type of component is likely.

In addition to the basic MAFO design just described, there are two specific designs that have been reported and are worthy of note. The first of these is the molded spiral AFO, as shown in Figure 7–9. This custom-molded device was developed by the Institute of Rehabilitation Medicine in New York and is often made of a semiflexible thermoplastic material called Nyloplex.[8] It is intended to provide resistance to both dorsiflexion and plantarflexion and is indicated primarily for a flail foot.

If the trimlines of the orthosis are such that they include a pretibial shell, the

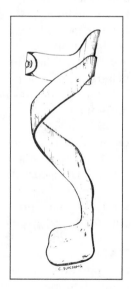

Figure 7–9. Molded spiral ankle-foot orthosis.

design is referred to as an anterior molded AFO or, sometimes, as a solid-ankle (SA) orthosis (Fig. 7–10). Usually the trimlines and thickness of the material result in a rigid ankle that is intended to prevent dorsiflexion of the ankle and/or knee flexion during the stance phase of gait, substituting for weak calf and/or quadriceps musculature. Because of its biomechanical effect of stabilizing the knee, this type of orthosis is sometimes referred to as a floor-reaction orthosis, (FRO).[9,10] Often it may be used with a soft heel and a rocker bar under the sole to simulate ankle motion.[11]

Weight-Bearing AFO

In some instances it may be desirable to limit the axial loading through the shank and foot. This goal can be accomplished through the use of a weight-bearing AFO, which is also frequently referred to as a patellar tendon-bearing orthosis.[12] This device (Fig. 7–11) uses the principles of weight bearing from the patellar tendon-bearing (PTB) prosthetic socket design to unload the skeletal structures below the knee. The axial forces are transmitted down the lateral uprights of the orthosis and the shoe to the ground. It has been reported that the weight-bearing function of the orthosis depends on variations in its design, on the amount of clearance between the heel and the inside of the shoe, and on the level of training the patient has received in its use.[13] When all of these factors are properly accounted for, up to 50% of a patient's weight can be borne through the orthosis during the entire stance phase. The design of the ankle joint is also an important factor in influencing how much force is transmitted to the orthosis. Often a rocker sole is used with these devices.

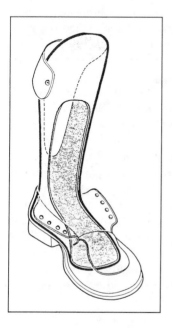

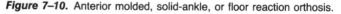

Figure 7–10. Anterior molded, solid-ankle, or floor reaction orthosis.

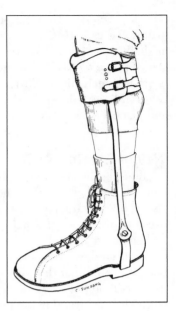

Figure 7–11. PTB Weight-bearing orthosis.

KNEE ORTHOSES

The three important functions of the knee during gait are shock absorption and support during stance and shortening during swing. Medio-lateral stability of the joint is assumed in healthy individuals but may be an important reason for applying an orthotic device to the knee. Similarly, a rotational derangement of the knee structures may necessitate the application of an external support. More recently knee orthoses (KOs) have been used prophylactically by athletes in an attempt to protect healthy knees from physical injury.[14]

If the problem is isolated to the knee joint, then only a KO should be used where possible. If other joints and structures are also involved, they need to be considered in selecting the appropriate orthotic design, as discussed in subsequent sections on knee-ankle-foot and hip-knee-ankle-foot orthoses. In many neuromusculoskeletal pathologies the support function of the knee joint may be inadequate. This may be due to insufficient neuromotor control, muscular weakness, or structural instability. The problem may manifest itself as a tendency toward excessive extension (ie, hyperextension); as a tendency toward insufficient extension, or knee buckling; or as excessive varus, valgus, or rotational instability. Additionally, a treatment goal may be to prohibit or at least limit knee motion to allow damaged or surgically repaired structures to heal. In all cases the reason for selecting and applying a particular orthosis should be clearly defined.

KOs comprise two types: solid-knee designs consisting of a rigid structure with no definable orthotic knee joint and articulating designs with a knee joint.

Rigid KO (Knee Cage)

The "Swedish" knee cage orthosis is a prefabricated device with a continuous metal piece making up the side bars and posterior cross member. The anterior thigh and calf straps are heavy elastic (Fig. 7–12). This device is intended for use in the prevention of mild genu recurvatum while providing some medio-lateral stability. The cosmesis of the device is considered to be poor, since the mediolateral dimension is bulky and the orthosis tends to protrude slightly when sitting.[15]

Molded Plastic Solid-Knee Orthosis

An orthosis similar in concept to the Swedish knee cage but custom fabricated of thermoplastic or plastic laminate materials is sometimes referred to as simply a solid-knee orthosis (SKO)[8]; (Fig. 7–13). Because it is custom made from a positive model of the limb, it can be expected to fit more intimately and to provide more precise control of the knee than an off-the-shelf knee cage. It has been recommended for mild-to-moderate genu recurvatum and is considered good cosmetically, although it does tend to protrude anteriorly when the patient is sitting, similarly to the Swedish knee cage. The Institute of Rehabilitation Medicine's single-piece design requires the device to be donned and doffed over the foot and leg, while the Nitschke bivalved design consists of two hinged halves.[16]

Extension KO

This device consists of two long, metal uprights with pivoting thigh and calf cuffs and an adjustable knee pad to provide gradual extension of the knee (Fig. 7–14). It is useful for correction of mild-to-moderate knee-flexion contractures with the knee pad being

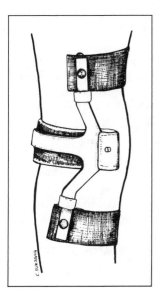

Figure 7–12. Swedish knee-cage orthosis.

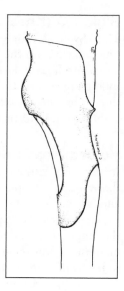

Figure 7–13. Molded-plastic SKO.

gradually tightened as correction occurs. It is sometimes used as a temporary orthosis to provide stabilization of the knee in the early stages of ambulation training.

Knee Immobilizer Orthoses

In many instances it is desirable to completely or nearly completely restrict motion of the knee. Often the restriction is only temporary to allow healing of damaged or surgically repaired internal structures. Sometimes, however, the need for restricted motion may be more permanent, as in the case of very weak or absent knee-extensor muscles, severe knee-joint deterioration, or hemophilia.

There are a number of prefabrication knee-immobilizer orthoses on the market that have a good deal of adjustability and can be expected to restrict knee motion reasonably well. These devices usually have several metal or plastic uprights incorporated into a fabric wrap. Some of the newer designs have rigid uprights attached to plastic shells with an orthotic knee joint to allow immobilization at positions of 0, 30, 60, or 90 degrees of knee flexion.

In contrast to off-the-shelf prefabricated knee immobilizers is the custom-fabricated molded-plastic knee immobilizer, sometimes referred to as a knee cylinder.[17] The orthosis consists of anterior and posterior sections that overlap medially and laterally and extend from just distal of the ischial tuberosity to just proximal of the malleoli. Suspension of the device is achieved by suprapatellar/supracondylar contouring. Because of its intimate fit, this device can be expected to distribute pressure evenly and to provide excellent restriction to knee movement, although no study is available to substantiate these expectations.

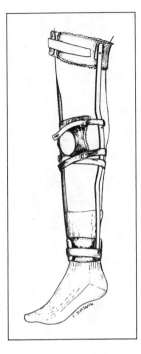

Figure 7–14. Extension KO.

Hinged-Knee Orthoses

A hinged-knee orthosis is sometimes also referred to as a hinged knee cage. The purpose of the device can be any one or a combination of the same purposes for applying knee orthoses without hinged joints, namely, to control or to prevent anteroposterior, mediolateral, or rotational instability or to reduce pain that may result from that instability.

A hinged-knee orthosis usually contains either plastic or metal uprights with SA or polycentric orthotic knee joints (Fig. 7–15). Additionally, the knee joints may include a locking mechanism, as described below in the section on knee-ankle-foot orthoses. The proximal and distal thigh and calf bands may be constructed of plastic, metal, leather, or fabric. Table 7–2 lists a number of KOs and the type of control reportedly provided by each.[18] A number of these devices and others have been described as derotation devices intended to protect or to support the knee against rotational instability. Some authors have claimed that some of these devices reduce strength and performance[19] while others have reported decreased instability from some designs.[20-22] For more information on any device, the reader is referred to the appropriate references at the end of the chapter and/or to the device manufacturer's literature.

In a series of 123 cases[23] fitted with a newer design of a hinged-knee orthosis, the most common indication for its use was postoperative protection for surgically repaired ligaments. The other large group of patients reported to have benefited from the device

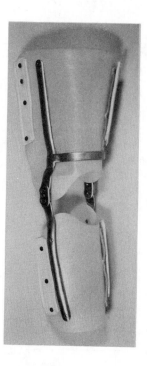

Figure 7–15. An example of a hinged KO, Iowa knee orthosis.

was the group with mediolateral instability secondary to chronic knee laxity. Other studies have reported on the prophylactic value of using such devices on collegiate football players as a means of preventing serious knee injuries.[14,24,25] Several cadaver studies have also provided information on the protection provided by various KOs against external forces.[26,27]

Telescoping KO

A device developed by the Canadian Arthritis and Rheumatism Society at the University of British Columbia[28] is intended for mediolateral stabilization of arthritic knees. The device consists of a plastic thigh and shank cuff attached to a telescoping tube by means of nylon joints. A knee cuff is located on the opposite side of the joint from the telescoping rod and provides the third pressure point for either medial or lateral stabilization of the knee, depending on how the device is applied. A waist belt is often used as an aid in suspending the orthosis.

KOs for Anteroposterior Instability

Most knee instability is due to medial or lateral collateral ligament injuries. For injuries in the anteroposterior plane, a different design of orthosis is often necessary. Marquette[29] has written a comprehensive review on the pathokinesiology of the injured knee. The four-strap configurations of the MKS II orthosis (Fig. 7–16) attempts to use the biomechanical principles developed by Marquette.

TABLE 7-2. COMPARISON OF PROPOSED FUNCTION OF VARIOUS KNEE ORTHOSES

Orthosis	Type of Control								
	Anteroposterior	Mediolateral	Collateral Ligament	Multiple Ligament	Rotatory	Recurvation	Patellar	Postoperative	Varus/Valgus
Generation II	X	X		X	X	X		X	
Lerman	X	X		X	X		X	X	
TRIO	X	X		X	X			X	
External Cruciate Ligament	X	X		X	X				
Can-Am	X	X			X				
Lenox Hill		X		X	X				
Iowa Knee Orthosis		X	X					X	
Anderson Knee Stabilizer		X	X						
Genucentric		X				X			
Teufel TKS		X				X			
CARS-UBC		X				X			X
Swedish Knee Cage						X			
Marshall-PAC							X		
Palumbo							X		

*Adapted from Beets CL, Clippinger FW, Hazard PR, Vaugh, DW. Orthoses and the dynamic knee: A basic overview. Orthot Prosthet. 1985; **39**(2):33–39.*

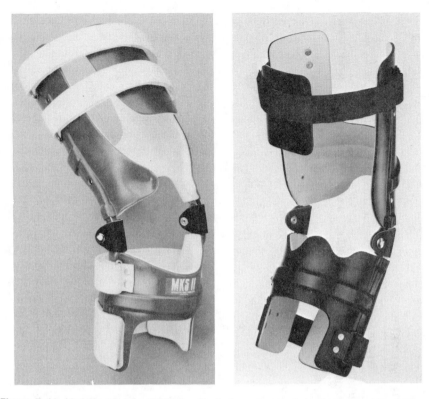

Figure 7–16. Variations of the MKS II orthosis for anteroposterior knee instability. (From Vixie Enterprises, Eugene, OR, with permission.)

Knee Wraps and Soft Supports

In addition to the devices mentioned above, there are a large number of knee wraps and soft supports that are available, principally for athletic and soft-tissue injuries. They are almost always prefabricated, off-the-shelf items that are used on a temporary basis.

KNEE-ANKLE-FOOT ORTHOSES

When an external device is required to augment function of both the foot-ankle and the knee, the device is referred to as a knee-ankle-foot orthosis (KAFO). Conceptually, KAFOs are a combination of KOs and AFOs. Sometimes an ankle-foot section is simply added to a KO as a means of suspending it or keeping it in place.

Single- and Double–Upright KAFO

The single- and double-upright KAFO can provide flexion and extension and mediolateral stabilization of the knee; it can also allow free, limited, or locked action at the ankle and/or knee. Dual upright KAFOs were formerly referred to as double long-leg braces or dual-channel long-leg braces. Molded plastic-hinged KAFOs consist of a MAFO joined to a plastic thigh cuff either by a metal or plastic composite knee joint. These molded plastic configurations offer the usual advantages of lighter weight and more intimate fit compared to metal and leather systems. A number of design variations are possible and often incorporate any one of a number of knee-locking mechanisms (Fig. 7–17).

A "free" orthotic knee joint provides no resistance to flexion and extension, although it may contain a stop or stops that limit the range of motion. A "drop" lock consists of a metal ring that slides down the superior section of the upright and encompasses an extension of the inferior section of the upright. When the patient fully extends the knee, gravity causes the ring to drop, preventing flexion of the knee until it is released by lifting upward. This type of lock functions similarly to the locked knee joints used in above-knee prosthetics. Often a spring-loaded rod or pullcord is attached to the drop-lock ring so that it can be lifted without having to reach down to knee level. Drop rings can be used on both medial and lateral uprights, but raising two drop rings simultaneously may be difficult. Davis[30] has reported on the development of a roller-bearing drop lock intended to reduce the amount of strength and dexterity needed to operate a drop-lock system. Another common type of an orthotic knee-locking mechanism is the Swiss, Schweitzer, or bail lock. This unit consists of a spring-loaded pin that locks the knee when it reaches full extension. The lock is released by pulling upward on a release lever. The release levers from both uprights are often connected by means of a metal "bail" looping around the posterior aspect of the knee. The wearer of the orthosis

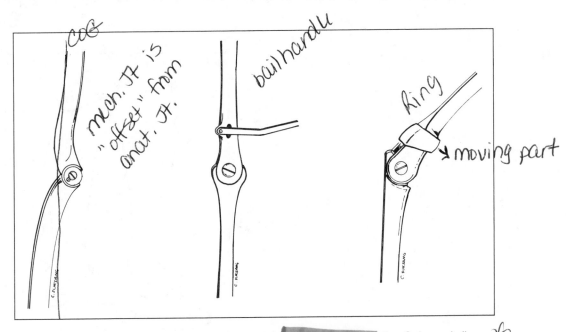

Figure 7–17. Examples of knee mechanisms: **left,** offset free knee; **center,** Swiss, or bail-handle lock; **right,** ring, or drop lock.

can open the locks by lifting the bail, usually by pressing it against a chair immediately before sitting.

Alignment of the orthotic knee joint is often crucial to the stability provided by the orthosis. Providing a posteriorly "offset" alignment to enhance knee stability is a common practice. The principles are similar to those used in above-knee prosthetic alignment, as discussed in Chapter 5. Double uprights can be expected to achieve better control of the limb than a single upright, but the increased bulk and weight of these components are important prescription considerations.

Supracondylar Shell KAFO

This device consists of either a dual-channel AFO or a molded-plastic AFO to which either a hinged or solid supracondylar shell has been added (Fig. 7–18). The supracondylar shell is intended to prevent excessive hyperextension of the knee while allowing full flexion. The design that does not have a knee joint poses a cosmetic problem when the wearer sits down. If the supracondylar cuff is very long, it will stick up noticeably.

Double-Bar Hip-Stabilizing KAFO

Another variation of the hinged KAFO is the double-bar hip-stabilizing orthosis (Fig. 7–19). This device was designed by personnel at the Craig Rehabilitation Institute specifically for the ambulatory management of patients with paraplegia.[31] Maximum knee and ankle stability is provided by a combination of offset locking-knee joints, locked ankle joints, and steel longitudinal stirrups in the soles of the shoes. The patient's legs are angled slightly forward, and he or she can lock the hips in the standing position by hip

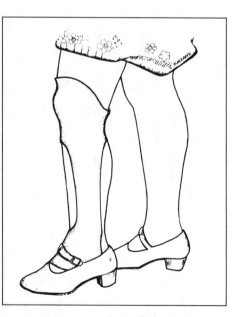

Figure 7–18. Supracondylar KAFOs.

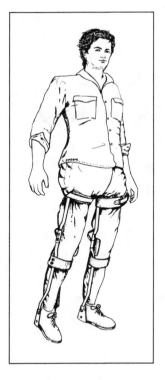

Figure 7–19. Double-bar hip-stabilizing KAFO.

hyperextension and lordosis. It is reported to be of value in the management of certain low-level paraplegics.

Quadrilateral Brim KAFO

At least partial axial unloading of the leg can be achieved by the use of a quadrilateral brim KAFO (Fig. 7–20). This device consists of a dual-upright or molded-plastic KAFO that has a thigh portion extending proximally to the ischial tuberosity and is configured similarly to a quadrilateral above-knee prosthetic socket. Effective weight bearing has been reported with this design, especially if a locked knee and ankle are used along with a rocker sole on the shoe.[13] Although total unloading of the skeletal structures is not possible, such a device can be useful in cases of structural deficiencies or in patients who have significant pain upon weight bearing.

Hip-Abduction KAFO

There are several design variations of hip-abduction KAFOs. Most of these devices have been used to treat Legg-Calvé-Perthes disease. (See also the following section.) Many designs, such as the one from the Toronto Crippled Children Center (Fig. 7–21)[32] and a similar device called the Newington orthosis,[33] allow full weight bearing with the use of crutches. The resulting gait pattern is understandably quite awkward and energy consuming.

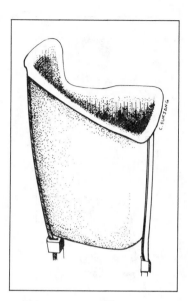

Figure 7–20. Quadrilateral brim KAFO.

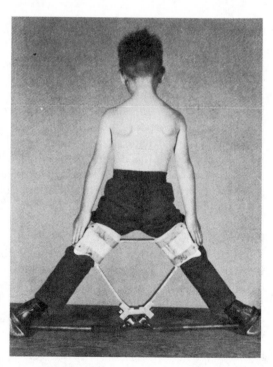

Figure 7–21. Example of a hip-abduction orthosis (Toronto).

HIP ORTHOSES

Besides unusual cases of severe trauma to the hip and pelvis, Legg-Calvé-Perthes disease is one of the principal problems requiring the application of hip orthoses. This self-limiting avascular necrosis of the epiphyseal center of the hip occurs primarily in males between the ages of 5 and 7 years and has been reported to require an average of approximately 20 months of orthotic management. The current containment theory of treatment attempts to maintain the affected hip in abduction and internal rotation for proper centralization of the femoral head within the acetabulum so that new bony growth will not be subjected to deforming forces.[34] In addition to the KAFOs mentioned above, the patient may be placed in a hip abduction orthosis, often referred to as the Scottish Rite orthosis[35] or a walking Lorenz (Fig. 7–22). This device features a pelvic band and hip joints with freely moving thrust bearings. The distal uprights of the joints are abducted 40 to 45 degrees and attach to thigh cuffs. Reported advantages of this device are that it is more conducive to active motion of the hip joints; has greater patient acceptability, since it can be easily worn under clothing; and appears to result in better patient compliance.[34]

A wide variety of hip abduction devices have been used in the treatment of congenital hip dysplasia. Allen[36] reported in 1962 on the complication of ischemic necrosis in patients treated with 90 degrees of hip abduction for hip dysplasia. Similarly, McCarroll[37] questioned the use of extreme hip-abduction positions and suggested that

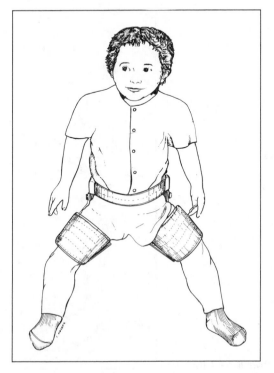

Figure 7–22. Scottish Rite orthosis for Legg-Calvé-Perthes disease.

they might contribute to increased interarticular pressure in the soft capital femoral epiphysis. Salter and Thompson[38] proposed replacing hip flexion and abduction with only hip flexion. Erlacher[39] reported on an orthosis developed in Czechoslovakia that maintains hip flexion angles of 90 to 110 degrees, allowing full abduction and adduction. Reportedly it allows active exercise within a specified hip flexion range, a feature thought by some to be an important component of treatment.

Orthotic devices have been used to control "scissoring" or spastic leg positions resulting from hypertonus of the hip adductor muscles. This problem is often seen in patients with cerebral palsy. A hip adduction-control orthosis is often worn at night to help prevent hip dislocation or subluxation and sometimes urinary disturbances.[40] Recently clinicians have used the Pavlik harness, positioning the hips in 110 degrees of flexion and 70 degrees of abduction (Weinstein S, personal communication, 1988).

HIP-KNEE-ANKLE-FOOT ORTHOSES

If a hip joint and pelvic band is added to a KAFO, the device is referred to as a hip-knee-ankle-foot orthosis (HKAFO; Fig. 7–23). The weight and cumbersomeness of these devices and the severity of involvement of patients requiring such an elaborate system make functional performance difficult. Patients' gaits in such systems are usually highly energy consuming, and four-point and swing-through assistive device patterns are

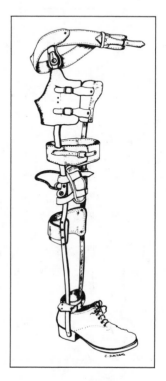

Figure 7–23. Conventional HKAFO.

usually required. Hoffer et al[41] reported on 56 patients with myelodysplasia using conventional HKAFOs in which only 35% of the patients could be considered household or community ambulators. In this study no patients with paralysis at the thoracic level became functional ambulators. The introduction of lightweight plastic components has improved this situation somewhat, and newer designs, such as the use of spring-extension assist hip joints, appear to offer improved chances of functional performance.[42]

The reciprocating gait orthosis (RGO) is a lumbosacral hip-knee-ankle-foot orthosis (LSHKAFO) developed to improve ambulation for patients with a myelodysplasia or dysfunctions of the hips and lower extremities (Fig. 7–24).[43] The key component of this system is a cable assembly that couples the flexion-extension motions of both hip joints. When the patient advances one lower extremity by flexion of the hip, the action of the cable assembly extends the contralateral hip. A cable release allows bilateral hip flexion for sitting. Many of the device components are made of polypropylene and aluminum to keep the orthosis as lightweight as possible. Studies by Yngve et al[44] and McCall and Schmidt[45] have reported reduced energy costs and increased walking speed with the RGO compared to ambulating with either locked or free hip joints. In the latter study all 41 of the patients with myelodysplasia preferred use of the reciprocating mode of the RGO. Thirty-four percent of the thoracic level, 70% of the upper lumbar level, and all of the lower lumbar level became community ambulators using the reciprocating gait orthosis.

A device often used in cases of lower-limb paralysis in children as a precursor to other orthotic systems or as a definitive device in itself is a rigid LSHKAFO, variously

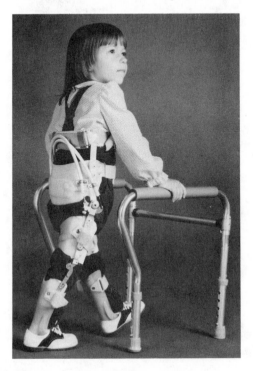

RGO - cables

Figure 7–24. Reciprocating gait orthosis. (Courtesy of Fillauer Orthopedic, Chattanooga, TN.)

referred to as a standing orthosis, swivel walker, or parapodium (Fig. 7–25).[46] These devices usually have a platform base attached to two or more uprights containing cuffs and/or straps. Little, if any, lower-extremity joint motion is allowed, since the device is intended to provide a rigid structure for maintaining the patient securely in an upright position rather than as an aid to functional ambulation. Some limited movement is possible by rocking the device from side to side and rotating the trunk and upper extremities.

FRACTURE ORTHOSES

Over the past 15 years or so there has been a progressive interest in the treatment of certain fractures of the lower limb by the use of orthotic devices, or "fracture braces," rather than the traditional plaster casts. The benefits to the patient include greater freedom of activity during the healing period, prevention of muscular atrophy and joint stiffness, shorter disability time, and apparent enhancement of the speed of fracture healing.[47] Some other possible advantages of using fracture orthoses compared to conventional plaster casts are that they allow the use of standard footwear, the patient can bathe regularly, the devices are lightweight, and the devices are easily removed so that open wounds can be cared for while boney alignment is maintained.

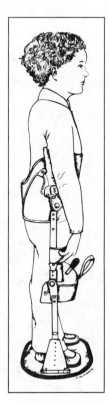

Figure 7–25. Parapodium.

Although many polypropylene off-the-shelf fracture orthoses are prescribed, many fractures are not straight and are not likely to fit into the prefabricated devices. In these cases a custom-molded fracture orthosis is the only means by which the goals of fracture healing can be attained.

OTHER LOWER-LIMB ORTHOSES AND MODIFICATIONS

Clearly not all possible lower-limb orthotic devices with all possible modifications and adaptations can be presented in a single chapter (or even in a single book). The devices described in this chapter have been included to familiarize the reader with many of the typical applications commonly seen in current orthotics practice. Regional differences and the preferences of particular orthotists and physicians mean that some of these devices will never be seen in certain locales and that other device variations not presented here will be regularly prescribed. In all cases, concerned, informed health care providers must communicate among themselves and with the patient to fully understand the goals for applying a particular device and keep abreast of the ever-evolving state of the art in lower-limb orthotics.

REFERENCES

1. *Rehabilitation Engineering Center. Lower limb Orthotics: A Manual.* Philadelphia, Pa: Moss Rehabilitation Hospital, 1978.
2. Perry J. Pathological gait. In: *Orthotics Atlas.* St. Louis, Mo: Mosby; 1975.
3. Glancy J. Orthotic control of ground reaction forces during running (A preliminary report). *Orthot Prosthet.* 1984; **38**(3):12–40.
4. McCollough NC. Current status of lower limb orthotics. *Orthop Dig.* 1975; 3:17–29.
5. Shurr D. Metal vs. plastic AFO—a therapist's view. *Clin Prosthet Orthot.* 1983; **7**(1):4.
6. Bensman A, Lossing W. A new ankle-foot orthosis combining the advantages of metal and plastics. *Orthot Prosthet.* 1979; **33**(1):3–10.
7. Showers D, David L. A reinforcing technique in orthotics and prosthetics. *Orthot Prosthet.* 1982; **32**(2):108–112.
8. Lehneis HR. New developments in lower limb orthotics through bioengineering. *Arch Phys Med Rehabil.* 1972; **53**(7):303–310.
9. Harrington E, Lin R, Gage J. Use of the anterior floor reaction orthosis in patients with cerebral palsy. *Orthot Prosthet.* 1983–1984; **37**(4):34–42.
10. Yang G, Chu D, Ahn J, Lehneis H, Conceicao R. Floor reaction orthosis: Clinical experience. *Orthot Prosthet.* 1986; **40**(1):33–37.
11. Glancy J, Lindseth RE. Solid ankle orthosis. *Orthot Prosthet.* 1972; **26**:14.
12. McIlmurray WJ, Greenbaum W. A below-knee weight-bearing brace. *Orthop Prosthet Appl J* 1958; **12**(2):81, 82.
13. Lehmann, JF. Lower limb orthotics. In Redford JB, ed. *Orthotics Etcetera* 3rd ed. Baltimore: Williams & Wilkins; 1975 p.317.
14. Randall F, Miller H, Shurr D. The use of prophylactic knee orthoses at Iowa State University. *Orthot Prosthet.* 1983; **37**(4):54–57.
15. *American Academy of Orthopaedic Surgeons, Orthotics Atlas.* St Louis, Mo: Mosby; 1975.

16. Nitschke RO, Marschall D. The PTS knee brace. *Orthot Prosthet.* 1968; **22**(3):46–51.

17. Pritham C, Stills M. Knee cylinder. *Orthot Prosthet.* 1980; **33**(4):11–17.

18. Beets CL, Clippinger FW, Hazard PR, Vaughn DW. Orthoses and the dynamic knee: A basic overview. *Orthot Prosthet.* 1985; **39**(2):33–39.

19. Houston M, Goemans P. Leg muscle performance of athletes with and without knee support braces. *Arch Phys Med Rehabil.* 1982; **63**(9):431–432.

20. Bassett G, Fleming B. The Lenox Hill brace in anterolateral rotatory instability. *Am J Sports Med.* 1983; **11**(5):345–348.

21. Knutzen K, Bates B, Hamill J. Electrogoniometry of post surgical knee bracing in running. *Am J Phys Med.* 1983; **62**(4):172–181.

22. Yelverton T, Pettersson G, Lysholm J, Gillquist J. The effect of derotation braces on knee motion. *Acta Orthop Scand.* 1988; **59**(3):284–287.

23. Shurr D, Miller H, Albright J, Feldick H. The Iowa knee orthosis. *Orthot Prosthet.* 1978; **32**(1):20–24.

24. Nicholas JA. Knee braces that protect against sports injuries. *J Musculoskel Med.* October 1986:56–61.

25. Hewson GF, Mendini RA, Wang JB. Prophylactic knee bracing in college football. *Am J Sports Med.* 1986; **14**(1):262–266.

26. Brown TD, Brand RA. Mechanical performance of prophylactic knee braces. Application for Research Grant (Orthopaedic Research and Education Foundation, Chicago, IL), September 1985.

27. Hofmann AA, Wyatt RWB, Bourne MH, Daniels AU. Knee stability in orthotic knee braces. *Am J Sports Med.* 1984; **12**(5):371–374.

28. Cousins D, Foort J. An orthosis for medial or lateral stabilization of arthritic knees. *Orthot Prosthet.* 1975; **29**(4):21.

29. Marquette S. A four-point stabilization for anterior-posterior knee control. *Orthot Prosthet.* 1988; **41**(4):18–26.

30. Davis L. An alternate system for locking the KAFO knee joint: A case study. *Orthot Prosthet.* 1985; **39**(2):61–64.

31. Hahn HR. Lower extremity bracing in paraplegics with usage follow up. *Paraplegia.* 1970; **8**(3):147–153.

32. Bobechko W, Mclaurin C, Motloch W. Toronto treatment in Legg-Perthes disease. *Art Limbs.* 1968; **12**(2):36–41.

33. Curtis B, Gunther S, Gossling, Paul S. Treatment for Legg-Perthes disease with the Newington ambulaton-abduction brace. *J Bone Joint Surg.* 1974; **56A**(6):1135–1146.

34. Pritham CH, Fillauer CE. Comtemporary trends in orthotic management of Legg-Calve-Perthes disease. *Orthot Prosthet.* 1985; **39**(1):62–69.

35. Purvis JM, Dimon III JH, Meehan PL, Lovell WW. Preliminary experience with the Scottish Rite Hospital abduction orthosis for Legg-Perthes disease. *Clin Orthop Rel Res.* 1980; **150**:49–53.

36. Allen RP. Ischemic necrosis following treatment of hip dysplasia. *JAMA.* 1962; **180**:497–499.

37. McCarroll HR. Diagnosis and treatment of congenital subluxation (dysplasia) and dislocation of the hip in infants. *J Bone Joint Surg.* 1965; **47A**:612.

38. Salter RB, Thompson GH. Legg-Calve-Perthes disease. *J Bone Joint Surg.* 1984; **66-A**(6):479–489.

39. Erlacher PJ. Early treatment of dysplasia of the hip. *J Int Coll Surg.* 1962; **38**:348–353.

40. Nakamura T. Ohamu M. Hip abduction splint for use at night for scissor leg of cerebral palsy patients. *Orthot Prosthet.* 1980; **34**(4):13–18.

41. Hoffer M, Feiwell E, Perry R, Perry J, Bonnett C. Functional ambulation in patients with myelomeningocele. *J Bone Joint Surg [Am].* 1973; **55**:137–148.

42. Brown J, Tindall G, Nitschke R, Haake P, Jackman K. Hip, knee, ankle foot orthosis: Lateral bar design with spring extension assist hip joints. *Orthot Prosthet*. 1982; **36**(4):44–49.

43. Douglas R, Larson P, D'Ambrosia R, McCall R. The LSU reciprocation-gait orthosis. *Orthopedics*. 1983; **6**(7):834–839.

44. Yngve D, Douglas R, Robert J. The reciprocating gait orthosis in myelomeningocele. *J Pediatr Orthop*. 1984; **4**:304–310.

45. McCall R, Schmidt W. Clinical experience with the reciprocal gait orthosis in myelodysplasia. *J Pediatr Orthop*. 1986; **6**:1157–1161.

46. Motlock W. The parapodium: An orthotic device for neuromuscular disorders. *Art Limbs*. 1971; **15**(2):36–47.

47. Mooney V, Nickel VL, Harvey JP, Snelson R. Cast-brace treatment for fractures of the distal part of the femur. *J Bone Joint Surg*. 1970; **52A**:1563–1578.

CHAPTER 8

Upper-Extremity Prosthetics

This chapter will address the incidence and etiology of upper-extremity amputations and the various levels at which they can occur. Further discussion will focus on upper-extremity prosthetic components, the operation and control of these prostheses, and the management of the upper-extremity amputee.

AN OVERVIEW OF UPPER-EXTREMITY PROSTHETICS

Although amputations of the upper extremity may be presumed to have occurred from very early times, the first record of an artificial device used for an upper-extremity amputation is thought to have come from the second Punic War, 218 to 201 BC. During that conflict Marcus Sergius, a Roman general, lost his right hand and was fitted with an iron hand that was reportedly used in battle with great dexterity. During the Middle Ages artificial limbs often appeared as part of a knight's suit of armor, serving to conceal any loss or disfigurement associated with battle.

Incidence

Malone et al[1] indicate that approximately 6,000 to 10,000 major amputations of the upper extremity occur every year in the United States. This does not include the numerous partial finger and thumb amputations that occur during work or recreation. In 1964 Glattly found approximately a 6-to-1 ratio of lower-extremity to upper-extremity amputations.[2] By 1975 the ratio had increased to approximately 11 to 1.[2] This ratio included both males and females and may be partly explained by a greater number of lower-extremity amputees rather than a smaller number of upper-extremity amputations. Kay and Newman[2] also found no change in the incidence of right- or left-sided amputations when compared with the Glattly study in 1964. Figure 1–2 (Chapter 1) depicts the amputation sites and compares the Glattly data with the 1975 data. Detailed data relative to the amputations of the upper extremity do not exist within the Kay and Newman[2] study and therefore cannot be further analyzed.

Etiology

Upper-extremity amputations occur for the same reasons that all amputations occur: trauma, tumor, disease, and congenital deficiencies.

Trauma. Although no comprehensive studies exist on the subject, trauma is undoubtedly the largest producer of upper-extremity amputations and can include fractures with or without lacerations; electrical and thermal burns; frostbite; and injuries from factory machines or tools and farm implements.

Tumor. The incidence of amputation caused by tumor varied little between 1964 and 1975 according to the two studies cited previously. Kay and Newman's[2] data demonstrate that approximately 4.5% of all the amputations of both lower and upper extremity may be attributed to tumors. Numerous accounts of the locations of primary bone tumors of the upper extremity reveal a large number occurring at proximal levels and at young ages (11 to 20 years). This is an unfortunate situation, since prosthetic devices for the upper extremity are much more functional and cosmetic when dealing with more distal sites of anatomic loss.

Disease. Unlike the lower extremity, peripheral vascular disease and diabetes do not play a major role in the etiology of amputations in the upper extremity. Since the blood flow to the upper extremity is greater in proportion to the lower extremity, it is far less common to see major limb amputations of the upper extremity done for vascular reasons. That is not to say, however, that they do not occur. In fact, it is very common to see patients with small-vessel disease secondary to diabetes, systemic lupus erythematosus (SLE), Raynaud's disease, or a number of other collagen-vascular diseases to have fingertips missing as a result of dry gangrene. These minor amputations do not require elaborate surgical procedures and rarely lead to functional restoration via prostheses.

Major limb amputations have been reported for vascular complications secondary to infections produced by drugs injected either into the back of the hand or into the web spaces of the digits. Because of the way the upper extremity is drained on the venous side, infection spreads rapidly. Lymphangitis and cellulitis can quickly overtake the limb, necessitating major surgical intervention and often amputation.

Other examples of upper-extremity amputations done for reasons of disease are those secondary to major episodes of sepsis, in which emboli are released, eventually occluding the major arterial tree of the arm and depriving the more distal components of their blood supply. These often occur following major episodes of sepsis in the very young when complications result from punctures of a major artery as part of treatment.

Congenital Deficiencies. Congenital limb deficiencies and amputations tend to occur more often in the upper extremity than in the lower. Unlike the counterpart congenital deficiency or amputation in the lower extremity, the primary purpose of any surgical revision or conversion in the upper extremity is to provide functional assistance and maintenance of sensation rather than conversion to a more standard level in preparation for prosthetic fitting and weight bearing. It is very important that such planned, or staged, surgical procedures not deprive the amputee of function or sensation necessary for activities of daily living, with or without prosthetic devices. As discussed in Chapter 10, certain specific problems exist in the congenital upper-extremity amputee, those being the preponderance of the left, short, below-elbow, terminal-transverse congenital amputation of the forearm and the statistical situation that describes the more common absence of three or four limbs if two limbs are affected.

Another factor specific to the congenital amputee is the phenomenon of bony overgrowth in which the appositional growth of the long bone exceeds the skin's ability to accommodate such growth and the bone actually pierces the skin, creating a wound, usually on the distal end of the stump. These are of no great sequelae and are treatable surgically by revision of the stump. Specifics relative to the phenomenon dealing with the actual bones and processes are described in Chapter 10 along with the differences between congenital amputations and deficiencies.

LEVELS OF UPPER-EXTREMITY AMPUTATION

Upper-extremity amputations are generally classified in two major categories: below-elbow and above-elbow amputations. As might be expected, there are important functional differences between having an intact elbow and a prosthetic elbow. Figure 8–1 depicts the various amputation levels of the upper extremity and includes the descriptive name usually given to each level.

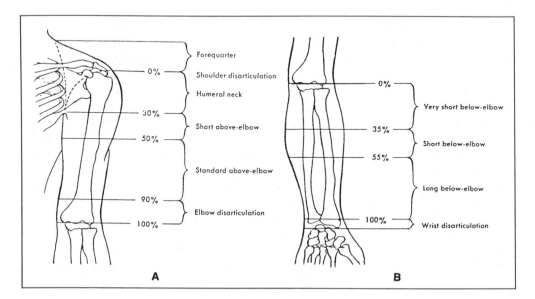

Figure 8–1. Upper-extremity amputation level; **(A)** above-elbow, **(B)** below-elbow. (From Kay HW, Newman JD. Relative incidences of new amputations *Orthot Prosthet.* 1975; **29**:8. with permission.)

Below Elbow

Partial Hand. Partial-hand amputations may be considered to be any number of amputations involving any or all of the digits or the radial or ulnar borders of the hand. These are, in fact, the most numerous amputations that occur in either the upper or lower extremity, but they usually require very little special postoperative treatment and/or prosthetic restoration.

Many articles and books have been written on the topic of partial-hand amputations and the surgical considerations relative to these injuries.[3,4] Partial-hand amputations are primarily produced by traumatic episodes that include fractures and soft-tissue injuries or both. It is important to realize that any traumatic injury to the hand may involve the nerves, robbing the hand of its ability to feel as well as to move. As the discussion of amputation and prosthetic restoration for upper-extremity amputations continues, the reader should be aware of the tremendous handicap produced by the absence or diminution of the sensory nerve supply, particularly to the palm of the hand and fingers, in the median nerve distribution.

An important element in the usefulness of any injured hand is the amount of function left in the thumb. Many staged operative procedures for partial-hand amputations are directed toward increasing the functional capabilities of the remaining parts, particularly the thumb and small finger, since opposition and holding usually require the border digits.

Wrist Disarticulation The wrist disarticulation-level amputation is usually performed when the partial-hand residual limb is without thumb or fingers and when the motion afforded by the wrist and palm of the hand has virtually nothing to oppose it. Very often the wrist disarticulation is not performed as a primary amputation but is done as an elective procedure after a patient discovers that a partial-hand prosthesis is cumbersome and not very functional.

According to Tooms,[5] a wrist disarticulation should allow normal distal-radial-ulnar joint motion, thus preserving pronation and supination (Fig. 8–2). Although approximately only 50% of the pronation-supination is transmitted to the prosthesis, wrist disarticulation remains the amputation of choice in situations where a long lever is advisable or important. Tooms[5] also recommends a long palmar flap, using the skin from the palm of the hand and the fascia under it to pad the distal stump. Burkhalter et al[6] indicate it is important that the radial and ulnar styloids be resected slightly to minimize the discomfort the amputee will endure in active pronation-supination within the confines of a hard prosthetic socket. Burkhalter comments on the scarcity of the true wrist-disarticulation amputation.[6] Several years ago, researchers at the University of Iowa Hospitals and Clinics attempted to find and recall all patients since 1930 who had undergone a wrist disarticulation. Upon searching 1.7 million medical records, only seven patients were identified as having true wrist-disarticulation operations.

Long Below-Elbow Amputation. According to Taylor,[7] a long below-elbow amputation is defined as one between 8 and 10 in from the center of the lateral epicondyle to the end of the residual limb. Reportedly this level allows the amputee to retain between

100 and 120 degrees of pronation-supination (Fig. 8–2). By allowing the amputee to use the long length of the residual limb as well as pronation-supination, this level provides an excellent opportunity for prosthetic restoration. Assuming a well-healed and equal lateral-flap closure, the long below-elbow amputation provides a functional residual limb for manual labor, farming, industrial work, and other similar occupations. It also provides good capability for lifting with the forearm.

Medium Below-Elbow Amputation. The medium below-elbow residual limb is defined as one between 6 and 8 in in length when measured from the lateral epicondyle. As can be seen from Figure 8–2, residual limbs significantly lose pronation-supination as they become shorter. At the medium below-elbow level, the amputee is well equipped to use standard prostheses to lift moderate weight with the forearm and to use the elbow without problems. Residual limbs of medium length allow the prosthetist considerable latitude in configuring the prosthesis. In some situations the prosthetist might wish to shorten the prosthetic limb compared to the contralateral side because of restricted range of motion of the elbow or shoulder. This level also lends itself to myoelectric or electric fittings, since the socket distal to the end of the residual limb has enough space to accommodate batteries and/or powered wrist units.

Short and Very Short Below-Elbow Amputation. Short and very short below-elbow amputations result in limbs between 2 and 4 in in length from the lateral epicondyle. In general, amputations at this length tend to present problems regarding suspension and

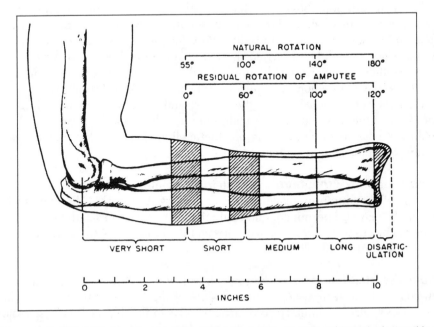

Figure 8–2. Rotation of residual forearm. (From Taylor CL. The biomechanics of control in upper extremity prosthetics. *Orthot Prosthet.* 1981; **35**:20, with permission.)

range of motion. Also of concern is the bunching of soft tissue in the anticubital fold anteriorly during elbow flexion beyond approximately 100 degrees. Many congenital limb deficiencies occur at the short and very short below-elbow level. These require special consideration due to the short length of the residual limb. In general, residual limbs below the elbow are more functional than an elbow disarticulation, assuming that the amputee has intact muscle power on both sides of the elbow joint. Short and very short residual limbs are usually held in a neutral position of pronation-supination for lifting, loading, and other functional activities.

Above Elbow

Elbow Disarticulation. There is little evidence in the literature to indicate that the additional length of the humerus is worth both the functional and cosmetic handicap associated with the elbow disarticulation-level amputation. In addition to the length, there is a problem of medio-lateral dimension, since the condyles of the distal humerus represent a large and bulky end that must somehow be included within a socket. Elbow disarticulation is a level usually reserved for children with growing epiphyses. A study by Shurr et al[8] shows that bony overgrowth in children tends to recur, necessitating multiple surgical procedures prior to skeletal maturity. For this reason amputation through the humerus should be avoided in children with open growth plates.

Long Above-Elbow Amputation. The long, or standard, above-elbow amputation is defined as one of 50% to 90% of the length of a normal humerus and is usually the level of choice for amputation above the elbow. With intact skin, musculature, and nerve supply to the arm, this length above-elbow amputation can provide the muscle power and range of motion necessary to produce very functional results with a conventional prosthesis. Since, as will be discussed shortly, glenohumeral flexion plays an important role in controlling a conventional body-powered system, the lever arm of the humerus allows the amputee excellent control over the device. This level may also produce excellent myoelectric signals from the biceps and triceps when operating a myoelectrically controlled system. Additionally, the prosthetist has a great deal of freedom in deciding at what level to place the prosthetic elbow joint and has easy access to the elbow unit for replacement or maintenance.

Short Above-Elbow Amputation. The short above-elbow amputation is defined as an amputation of the humerus leaving 30% to 50% of its length. Although such short residual limbs may still permit adequate functioning of a prosthesis, the lack of length of the humerus places some serious constraints on the placement of the control cables used to operate the prosthetic elbow.

Shoulder Disarticulation. The shoulder disarticulation (SD) may be defined as any amputation of the arm from approximately 30% of the humerus through the shoulder joint. In cases where the humerus is disarticulated completely, there is no question that prosthetically the amputation results in a shoulder-disarticulation level. However, in those cases where there is a remaining bit of humerus, functionally the patient will be a prosthetic candidate for a shoulder-disarticulation prosthesis even though he or she is anatomically not a true shoulder-disarticulation amputee. Considering the anatomy, the patient may have up to 30% of the length of the upper humerus but have little motor power available in flexion, extension, or abduction. Therefore a prosthetic shoulder joint must be considered. As is the case in regard to the hip in the lower extremity, shoulder-disarticulation amputations are often performed for reasons of tumor. It is indeed unfortunate that the tumor invades the limbs near their upper junctions with the body, necessitating many prosthetic joints and large and often bulky prosthetic sockets.

Forequarter Amputation. The most proximal level of amputation surgery in the upper extremity is referred to as the forequarter. Like the shoulder disarticulation, it is usually performed because of a tumor. In the forequarter the clavicle and scapula are usually sacrificed as well as the entire length of the humerus and the rest of the arm. In addition, various lengths of ribs may be sacrificed, depending on the nature of the tumor and the reconstruction goals of the surgeon. If the scapula is removed on the amputated side, the range of bilateral scapular abduction is diminished by one half. As will be seen, this motion is important when body-powered systems are used to operate a prosthetic arm. The forequarter amputation would appear to be an ideal level for using an externally powered prosthesis. However, systems used at the forequarter level are fraught with difficulties because of the restricted number of motor sites available for myoelectric signal pickup. Careful attention to detail on the part of the surgeon is necessary at this level so that no bony prominences remain under compromised skin. This situation can lend itself to many problems in fitting the very large socket that often encompasses part of the sound-side shoulder in an attempt to minimize the tendency for the socket to rotate and fall off.

COMPONENTS OF UPPER-EXTREMITY PROSTHESES

Prosthetic components in the upper extremity are analogous to components in the lower extremity. A below-elbow prosthesis consists of a socket, a spacer or prosthetic extension, and what is generically referred to as a terminal device, typically a hook or prosthetic hand. In the case of an above-elbow prosthesis, there is an additional prosthetic extension and an elbow unit. A shoulder-disarticulation or forequarter prosthesis may also contain a shoulder joint. In this section we will discuss terminal devices, below-elbow and above-elbow sockets, elbow units, and shoulder-disarticulation prostheses. Techniques commonly used to activate terminal devices and to control prosthetic elbows using both body-powered and externally powered systems will be presented in the following section.

Partial-Hand Prostheses

Partial-hand prostheses are relatively uncommon, and although books from the time of Bunnell[4] to Bender[3] contain many partial-hand, nonstandard prostheses and hooks, these devices are often abandoned as time passes and the amputee grows accustomed to life with something other than a normal hand. Exceptions occur when the amputee is bilaterally involved or when the amputee's occupation or vocation can only be accomplished through the use of such a device.

Terminal Devices

A terminal device is a component used to produce holding or prehension and may be either a hook, hand, or nonstandard device. Terminal devices (TD) are usually interchangeable, applied using a threaded connector. They are either made of stainless steel or aluminum, may be covered with neoprene or plastizol, and are available in numerous designs. Stainless-steel TDs weigh more than aluminum, and the level of prosthetic restoration may dictate the type of TD prescribed. The shorter the above-elbow level, the more necessary it is to use a lightweight, aluminum TD. Amputees returning to heavy industrial or farm work usually require stainless steel TDs. In a device described as voluntary opening (VO), biscapular abduction opens the terminal device, and rubber bands close it as the abduction is reduced. Voluntary closing (VC) devices work just the opposite but are far less prevalent.

Hosmer/Dorrance is the name usually associated with conventional TDs. These TDs are named by numbers, in reverse order of size, with 3 being the largest and heaviest and 12 the smallest and lightest. Hooks may be either canted or lyred in shape. Canted fingers permit better visualization of the object in the TD. The "thumb" of the TD is where the control cable attaches and is the point where the opening force is applied (Figure 8–3).

Hands. Prosthetic hands may be either body powered or electric. Hands are interchangeable with hooks by means of a hook-to-hand adaptor. Electric hands may be either myoelectrically controlled or switch controlled. Myoelectric control is thought to be the most natural and normal. Body-powered hands are voluntary opening and spring closed. Pronation and supination are accomplished by prepositioning using the sound hand and are maintained by friction in the wrist unit.

Nonstandard Terminal Devices. An example of a nonstandard TD is the Greifer from Otto Bock. This TD is plastic covered and is used with electric prostheses. Disadvantages of this type of TD are increased weight, reduced cosmesis, and unavailability for small women or children.

Hook Versus Hand. Various studies are available dealing with the issue of hooks *v* hands. Hooks are generally believed to produce superior prehension compared to hands, particularly when picking up small objects. Hands produce only palmar prehension and are not as effective with smaller objects. Hands are generally thought to be more cosmetic, although one could certainly question the "cosmesis" of a functionless, motionless hand.

Sorbye,[9] a psychologist from Sweden, advocates self-suspending, self-contained, myoelectrically controlled below-elbow prostheses for children. He believes that children should be fitted between the ages of 2½ and 4 years of age. He had been successful in developing a child-sized hand, which was not available previously. Studies by Hagg et al[10] indicate children open and close these prostheses 2000 to 3000 times per day.

Children under 1 year of age have been fitted with myoelectric prostheses. What remains unclear is whether there is an advantage to myoelectric fittings and whether functionally these children grow up to be better wearers and users than their counterparts fitted at similar ages using conventional, body-powered components.

Trost[11] reported on 47 children fitted with myoelectric prostheses between the ages of 6 and 16 years, averaging 12.5 years. All had been previously fitted with a conventional prosthesis. Sixteen of 47 rejected the prostheses due to lack of durability, poor function, and increased weight. Advantages shared by these 16 were lack of a harness, ease of operation, and comfort. Trost recommended fitting children at ages 9 to 11 years with myoelectric prostheses.

Northmore-Ball et al[12] reported on 43 traumatic workmen, who were fitted with both conventional and myoelectric control. The data concluded that in social engagements these amputees wore the myoelectric arm 91% of the time; but during work only 15% used the myoelectric arm for fear of damaging the prosthesis.

In a study by Stein and Waller,[13] 36 upper-extremity amputees, 20 with myoelectric control and 16 with conventional prostheses, performed tasks with both arms, comparing both with a normal hand. Results indicated that the tasks took five times longer than normal using the myoelectric prosthesis. These tasks were performed two times faster using conventional control compared with myoelectric. Stein also reported that conventional users will use the hook only when it can be done quickly, otherwise they prefer the hand. He concluded that 60% of the below-elbow amputees preferred the myoelectric control and hand.

Below-Elbow Components

A common prescription for a below-elbow amputee resuming some type of industrial or heavy labor may include a total-contact socket with single-pivot elbow hinges and triceps cuff (Fig. 8–3).

Conventional Socket. Although upper-extremity prosthetic sockets are not end bearing or even weight bearing, the need for total contact demands a snug, intimate fit around the residual limb. A conventional double-wall socket includes the lamination of the socket itself plus a second lamination pulled over the first to provide cosmesis, stability, and function. During the casting phase of the fabrication process, the prosthetist pays careful attention to the distribution of pressure around and including the epicondyles, the contact with cut bones, and the olecranon. Adequate relief in the anterior distal socket must be given to the radius so that lifting will not cause high levels of pressure and pain. Attention is also given to the posterior portion of the socket so that lifting will not cause undue pressure on the olecranon. The trimlines of the below-elbow socket depend a great deal on the length of the residual limb. The shorter the residual limb the higher or more proximal the trimlines; the longer the residual limb the lower the trimlines. Another consideration for trimlines includes the desire to allow pronation and supination. A high anterior trimline will not allow pronation-supination to occur at the radial ulnar joint of the forearm.

If the terminal device of the prosthesis is ultimately to be positioned near the mouth and if the amputee has restricted range of motion at the elbow, the prosthetist

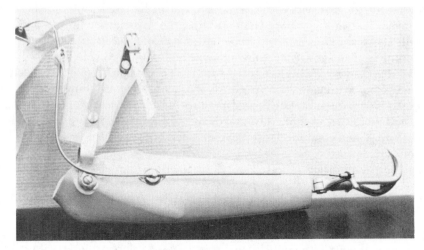

Figure 8–3. Standard below-elbow SA hinges, triceps cuff, TD.

may install the prosthesis in an attitude or angle of preflexion. This preflexion is a combination of the normal hanging angle, or the 10 to 15 degrees in which the elbow normally flexes, coupled with any additional flexion necessary to reach the mouth. Often the wrist unit may be slightly canted in an antero-medial direction to assist the amputee in getting the terminal device to the midline.

Elbow Hinges. Single-pivot stainless steel hinges are used when heavy-duty use is anticipated. Since the suspension of the prosthesis is handled primarily by the harness, there is little need to develop an auxiliary suspension on the condyles around the elbow. This allows the amputee full use of the elbow joint in an attempt to gain whatever elbow range of motion possible. Although stainless steel single-pivot hinges are very durable, they also eliminate pronation-supination. In contrast, flexible hinges are designed to maintain the available pronation-supination to avoid prepositioning of the terminal device using the normal hand. The classic application for flexible hinges is at the level of wrist disarticulation, where the patient theoretically has full pronation-supination available and a good long lever with which to not only flex the elbow but also pronate and supinate the terminal device. In some cases, however, the amputee is not able to tolerate the forces generated by the prosthesis on the residual limb. These forces are often eliminated and absorbed by rigid hinges.

Muenster Socket. The Muenster, or Hepp-Kuhn self-suspending, socket was originally developed for congenital below-elbow amputees to be used with passive cosmetic hands in short and very short below-elbow amputations. The prosthesis was meant to be a light-duty prosthesis, often used for females, adolescents, or myoelectric fittings. Contraindications therefore included residual limbs longer than 5 ½ in, the desire to use pronation and supination, amputees requiring heavy-duty lifting, or bilateral amputees.

To suspend the Muenster socket, pressure is exerted proximally in an anteroposterior direction by the prosthetist during the casting phase. In conjunction with a higher cubital-fold trimline, this pressure produces forces on the olecranon and the area in the cubital fold surrounding the biceps tendon. In longer residual limbs, pressure is applied distally and anteriorly around the biceps tendon. There is virtually no compression or suspension generated by the epicondyles of the humerus. A limitation in elbow flexion is inherent in the original Muenster design. The shorter the residual limb the higher the trimline anteriorly and the less range of motion available to the amputee. Variants using epicondyle suspension as well as posterior olecranon cutouts have been developed by Sauter and others in an attempt to alleviate some of the difficulties caused by the restricted range of motion in the original Muenster design (Fig. 8–4).

The Split Socket. In cases where a conventional below-elbow or Muenster-type socket is not possible and in cases where either limited range of motion or limited available muscle power creates problems with elbow flexion, other options exist. The split socket (Fig. 8–5) consists of a socket within a socket, attached by either step-up or variable-gear elbow hinges. These hinges use gear ratios to produce flexion of the prosthesis that is greater than flexion of the elbow joint, often by a factor of two. In a case where the amputee has only 60 degrees of active elbow flexion, a geared hinge or variable step-up hinge enables the amputee to develop 120 degrees of elbow flexion, thus enabling him or her to bring the terminal device to the mouth. The prosthesis is often a bit uncosmetic and demands a force factor of two times normal in exchange for the added elbow range of motion. Additionally, the control of the forearm section and terminal device of such a prosthesis may be difficult, and lifting may be contraindicated, since objects falling out of the grasp of the terminal device will propel the forearm section toward the midline uncontrolled, in some cases hitting and/or injuring the patient.

Stump-Activated Locks and Fair-Lead Controls. If an amputee cannot maintain a desired angle of elbow flexion, a stump-activated elbow lock is available. This lock

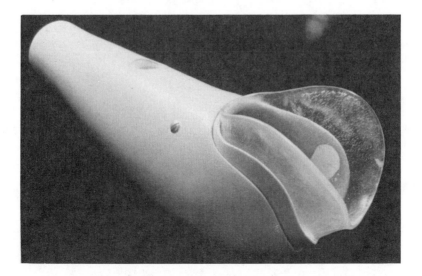

Figure 8–4. Otto Bock flexible acrylic supracondylar suspension.

allows the patient to develop the appropriate amount of flexion and then to lock the hinge at the desired position. Lock activation usually requires motion of the triceps muscles.

In cases where an amputee is unable to produce enough power to flex the elbow, a split-housing system or fair lead similar to that used in above-elbow prosthetics may be used. This allows a pull on the cable, usually using biscapular abduction, to flex the elbow until approximately 100 degrees of elbow flexion occurs. The elbow is then locked, and further pull on the cable opens or closes the terminal device, similar to many above-elbow systems. It is important to understand that the prostheses in this section are used very infrequently and only in cases where both patient and prosthetist known that severe tradeoffs in force and excursion exist and that complete range of motion and terminal device opening may be compromised no matter what prosthetic restoration is provided.

Above-Elbow Components

The Above-Elbow Socket. Although the above-elbow socket does not bear weight or even accommodate axial load, it is important that the socket be well fitted. The trimlines of the above-elbow socket are a function of the length of the residual limb. For a standard-length above-elbow residual limb, the lateral trimline should cross the proximal acromion. The anterior trimline borders the deltopectoral groove, and the posterior trimline borders the scapula. In the short above-elbow amputation, the lateral trimline should include the acromioclavicular joint, the anterior trimline should include the deltopectoral groove, and the posterior trimline should include 1 in of the remaining scapula. Conceptually the trimlines for the short above-elbow prosthesis will cover the acromioclavicular joint to assist in suspension and cover the deltopectoral groove and scapula in the anterior and posterior portions in an effort to control rotation.

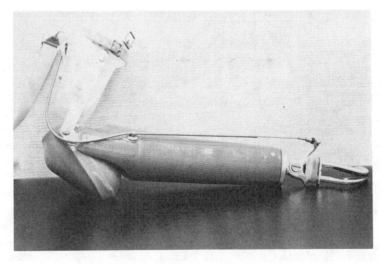

Figure 8–5. The split socket with step-up hinge.

The medial wall of the above-elbow socket is flattened so that it lies comfortably against the chest (Fig. 8–6). The anterior wall must contour the residual limb while allowing relief for the cut end of the humerus. Since glenohumeral flexion is used to flex the elbow and open and close the terminal device, it is very important that no undue pressure be allowed on the cut end. Although the lateral and posterior walls primarily cover soft tissue, it is important that they contour exactly the patient's remaining anatomy. The socket must be tight fitting but at the same time not restrictive. A total contact socket retards swelling of the limb and provides good proprioception relative to the position of the arm and shoulder. Upon inspection of the socket, the medial and lateral dimensions will look relatively flat, while the anterior and posterior walls will appear slightly rounded in part because of the bulk of the musculature and the attempt to restore the normal-looking anatomy of the biceps and triceps.

Elbow Units. Flexion of the elbow is simulated by rotation of the turntable component of the elbow unit, which allows the amputee to preposition the forearm relative to the body without changing the neutral position of the above-elbow socket. Since most standard above-elbow amputations are between 50% and 90% of the length of the humerus, it is possible to use the internally locking elbow as the main component of body-powered above-elbow prostheses. In most cases, assuming reasonable muscular control and skin coverage, this provides a very functional level with which to drive the above-elbow prosthesis. The shorter the length of the humerus and the shorter the position of the base plate and retainer the more difficult to develop excursion of the cable and therefore the more difficult to perform activities that occur with the elbow flexed and the terminal device open, usually near the patient's midline or mouth. Although full terminal-device opening is not a goal of most unilateral above-elbow amputees, it remains a goal for many patients, even though one normal hand remains. Patients with short above-elbow amputations have difficulties performing full terminal-

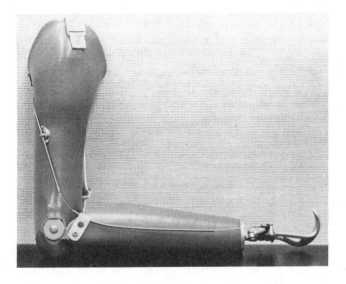

Figure 8–6. Above-elbow socket.

device opening near the mouth. In cases where myoelectric control is desired, the standard-length above-elbow amputation provides an excellent source of myoelectric signal pickup using the biceps anteriorly and the triceps posteriorly.

Externally Powered Elbows. There are currently several externally powered elbows commercially available. These are the Hosmer NYU, the Boston elbow, and the Utah arm. These elbows may either be myoelectric or switch controlled and are now interchangeable using the myoelectric hands. It should be well understood that patients desiring this sophisticated equipment are not seen often in a general prosthetic practice but are often referred to prosthetists who have an interest in such cases and who have taken the time to learn the circuitry and components well.

Because of the limitations imposed by the design, cost, maintenance, and down time, many prosthetists use hybrid systems, using a conventional, body-powered elbow and a myoelectrically controlled hand. Much credit should be awarded to a few individuals worldwide who have pioneered the practice of upper limb, myoelectrically controlled prostheses. Among those names are Schmidl of Italy; Billock, Jacobsen, LeBlanc, and Childress of the United States; Sorbye of Sweden; Herberts of Denmark; Hepp, Kuhn, Marquardt, and Biedermann of West Germany; and Sauter of Canada.

Shoulder-Disarticulation Components. As mentioned previously, the prosthesis for a very short above-elbow amputation is virtually identical to a shoulder-disarticulation prosthesis, since the length of the humerus is such that it cannot functionally generate useful motion. Available motions for operating the terminal device and/or elbow unit include shoulder elevation and depression as well as biscapular abduction. For all practical purposes, glenohumeral flexion is not available at this level. The socket, of necessity, covers the acromion and scapula and must include relief for these bony prominences (Fig. 8–7). The socket may be referred to as a shoulder cap in that it covers the shoulder, allowing no motion yet suspending the socket by long trimlines anterior, superior, and posterior. The axillary component is similar to an above-elbow socket in that it must allow easy entry yet a snug fit with minimal superior displacement.

It is more difficult to generate excursion of control cables as the length of the humerus shortens. Therefore short above-elbow or shoulder-disarticulation amputees have great difficulties activating their prostheses. Single glenohumeral flexion is no longer available, biscapular abduction needs to provide the motor power for flexion of the elbow as well as opening of the terminal device. To assist with elbow flexion, an elbow-flexion assist (Fig. 8–8) or a spring-loaded device mounted on the medial side of the prosthetic elbow may be used allowing the prosthetist to move the elbow-flexion attachment closer to the elbow center. This captures additional excursion necessary for terminal-device opening in full-elbow flexion.

From a functional point of view it must be emphasized that the very short above-elbow and shoulder-disarticulation amputees will use their prostheses only for assistance or specific tasks. It is difficult to expect body-powered above-elbow prostheses to significantly contribute to such activities of daily living as feeding and dressing. Currently patients with good abilities to biscapularly abduct and shoulder flex can be fitted with body-powered elbows and myoelectrically controlled hands. This "hybrid" combi-

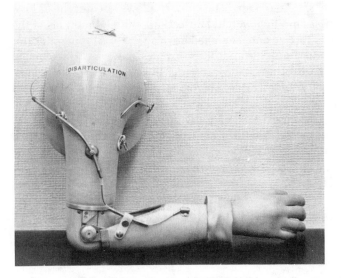

Figure 8–7. Shoulder-disarticulation prosthesis.

nation seems to address the needs of both the patient and the prosthetist in that the present state of the art makes it very difficult to use an electric elbow and myoelectric hand in the same prosthesis.

Forequarter Components. Different from the shoulder disarticulation, the forequar-ter amputation requires a more extensive socket usually covering part or all of the sound-side shoulder. The socket on the involved side is also longer and larger than in shoulder disarticulation or above-elbow levels. Sauter from Canada developed a fitting

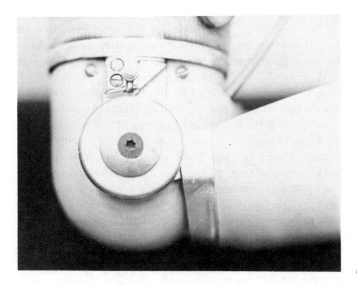

Figure 8–8. Elbow-flexion assist.

frame instead of a solid-plastic shoulder cap. This frame allows greater heat loss, excellent cosmesis and suspension, and lightweight fabrication. With all motions of the shoulder gone, available force production and excursion are also gone. Amputees at this level require at least an excursion amplifier and often external power. An excursion amplifier is a pulley system geared on a ratio of 2:1. As the amputee pulls 1 in of excursion, the amplifier delivers 2 in of cable movement. The price paid for this excursion is force in that it requires a double amount of force to produce the 2-in excursion. Harnessing may be customized to each individual patient's needs. Motions available include chest expansion or shoulder elevation. Switches may be incorporated into the chest expansion or shoulder elevation system to turn on electric motors driving either the elbow or the terminal device if myoelectric controls are not possible. The forequarter needs to be as lightweight and cosmetic as possible. After fitting it is not uncommon for many patients to reject the prosthesis and to opt for a shoulder cap made of plastic and foam that effectively fills the shirt or blouse while providing a useful function.

OPERATION AND CONTROL OF UPPER-EXTREMITY PROSTHESES

Sources of Body Power

Nonelectric prostheses require body power through harnessing of available motions to produce desired prosthetic control or function. Several options are available throughout the upper extremity and thorax. In body-powered, cable-driven artificial limbs, two concepts underlie the use of functional body power. These two concepts are force and length. Force is necessary to pull on a cable to produce functioning of the prosthesis. Length is important, since it will determine the extent of the resulting motions at the elbow and hand.

Whether an above-elbow or below-elbow amputation, perhaps the best overall movement with regard to both force and length is glenohumeral flexion. Taylor[7] states that between 40 and 60 lb of force can be generated by the average adult in glenohumeral flexion. This is more than enough to operate and control above- or below-elbow prostheses. In addition to force, glenohumeral flexion produces good length and may be harnessed easily, depending on the length of the humerus.

Another excellent source of body power is shoulder elevation/depression. Shoulder elevation/depression is used primarily for locking and unlocking elbows in short above-elbow, shoulder-disarticulation, or forequarter-length amputations. Although shoulder elevation produces good force and good length, it requires a fixed point, usually at the waist, to provide an anchor against which to pull. This anchor often is movable if connected to either a belt or pants. A more secure means of using shoulder elevation is by means of a peroneal strap or strap that goes through the groin on the opposite side of the amputated shoulder. However, peroneal straps are very uncomfortable for most patients and are not tolerated except by very short, bilateral, usually amelic, children.

Scapular abduction or protraction produces a good force with which to operate the terminal device or to flex the elbow of a prosthesis. Studies have indicated that 2 in of cable excursion is needed to open and close a terminal device with the elbow in neutral.

Although the force produced by scapular abduction is good, its length is limited. However, when both scapula are available, the required 2 in usually can be accomplished.

Shoulder depression may be used, since it produces a good force but restricted length. Shoulder depression is often harnessed to produce the required ⅝ to ¾ in excursion needed to lock or unlock the elbow of an above-elbow prosthesis.

Chest expansion is another motion that may be used because of its good force but only moderate excursion. Chest expansion is often used to lock or to unlock the elbow of a shoulder-disarticulation or forequarter-level amputation.

Combinations of the aforementioned motions may be used in specific situations. For example, in congenital amputees, locks of either elbow or shoulder may be accomplished by residual dysplastic hands, particularly ones located in nonanatomic places. Such conditions as phocomelia may also lend themselves to nonstandard applications.

Below-Elbow Harnessing

The harness of choice for the below-elbow amputee is a figure-8 harness and a Northwestern ring. Figure 8–9 demonstrates the figure-8 harness from both the anterior and posterior perspectives. The components of the below-elbow harness include the axillary loop, which serves as an anchor for the terminal device to pull against; the anterior suspensor strap lying in the deltopectoral groove on the involved side and maintaining the primary suspension of the prosthesis; and the control attachment strap originating on the ring and lying on the lower third of the scapula, incorporated into the hanger and the cable. The ring lies flat on the back, inferior to C-7 and just to the sound side of the center of the spine. It is important that the harness be tight enough to activate the

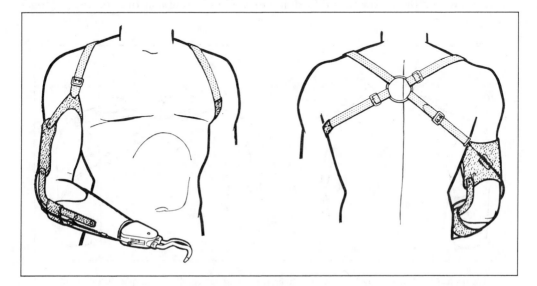

Figure 8–9. Figure-8 harness.

terminal device and loose enough to be comfortable and to allow the amputee freedom of movement of both arms and both shoulders. As was noted previously, the primary motor source for the below-elbow figure-8 harness is glenohumerous flexion. An increase in the angle of glenohumeral flexion will open the terminal device; the rubberbands will close it as the amputee extends the elbow. In the case where the amputee desires to open the terminal device close to the body, biscapular abduction is used. Adduction or retraction is used to allow the split hook to return to its closed position.

Above-Elbow Harnessing

The harness of choice for the above-elbow prosthesis is a figure-8 harness with a sewn crosspoint located inferior to C-7 and to the sound side (Fig. 8–10). These components are similar to the figure-8 harness used at the below-elbow level with the addition of the anterior suspensory strap and the elbow-lock cable strap mounted to the anterior suspensor strap. The anterior suspensory strap is composed of two parts, the dacron strap running posteriorly to anteriorly over the shoulder and into the delto-pectoral groove. One inch inferior to the clavicle this dacron strap is connected to a piece of elastic webbing that terminates at the distal and slightly medial portion of the humeral component of the prosthesis. This acts to return the elbow-lock cable after each pull. A dacron strap located more superficial to the elastic strap activates the elbow lock. It is important that the axillary loop on the above-elbow harness remains tight and consistent in its location in the sound-side axilla. This acts as the anchor from which the other two straps pull.

Standard above-elbow harnessing requires certain motor functions. Those motor sources are biscapular abduction and glenohumeral flexion. Biscapular abduction opens and closes the terminal device with the elbow locked and flexes and extends the elbow when it is unlocked. Studies at New York University indicate that it requires 2 in of excursion to flex the elbow to full flexion and 2½ in of excursion to open the terminal

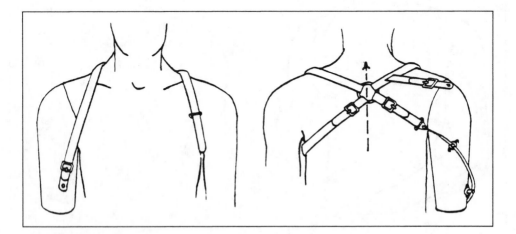

Figure 8–10. Above-elbow harness. (From Northwestern University Prosthetic Orthotic Center, 1987, with permission.)

device fully at the mouth. Therefore a total of 4½ in of excursion is necessary to fully operate an above-elbow prosthesis. A combination motion of shoulder depression, abduction, and extension produces ⅝ to ¾ in of excursion and 2 lb of force to activate the elbow-locking cable.

The above-elbow control system is termed dual control, although it also has two cables. Dual control refers to the concept of one cable flexing and extending the elbow and, when locked, also opening and closing the terminal device. To produce flexion of the elbow, the cable passes slightly anterior to the elbow hinge. The housing through which the cable runs is discontinuous and sometimes referred to as a fair lead. With the elbow unlocked, this fair lead allows the pull on the cable to flex the elbow, pulling the two housings together at the elbow. As was indicated previously, it requires approximately 2.5 in of cable excursion to flex the elbow. The distal housing, from the elbow center to wrist unit, is connected to the forearm by a component called an elbow-flexion attachment. This elbow flexion attachment controls the position of the cable relative to the elbow joint. It allows for adjustment by the prosthetist to provide the most optimum terminal device function. The more distal the location of the elbow-flexion attachment the less force that is required to flex the elbow, since the perpendicular distance from elbow center is increased. This also results in a need for greater excursion. On the other hand, moving the elbow-flexion attachment more proximal to the elbow center demands more force to flex the elbow but uses less excursion. Since most normal above-elbow amputees have no problem generating force and often have problems generating excursion, proximal location of the elbow flexion attachment may be advantageous.

MANAGEMENT OF THE UPPER-EXTREMITY AMPUTEE

Preoperative Care

Although a smaller number of upper-extremity amputations are done on an elective basis compared with the lower extremity, it is good practice for the clinic team members to visit with the elective upper-extremity amputee before the surgical procedure. Many of the questions and concerns discussed in Chapter 1 are of concern to the upper-extremity patient. In many cases the patient's questions deal with the timing of certain procedures and the availability of prosthetic restoration with or without "bionics."

Postoperative Care

As with lower-extremity amputees, postoperative programs for upper-extremity amputation include exercise, compression wrapping, and provision of preparatory prostheses.

Exercise. Depending on the level of amputation, the muscles about the joint proximal to the amputation must be mobilized and exercised as early as medically possible. These exercises will prevent the negative effects of disuse and will allow the amputee good use of muscles and joints in preparation for prosthetic restoration. Specifically, below-elbow patients need to emphasize elbow flexion and primarily elbow extension. They also must not forget the muscles about the shoulder, particularly the abductors and external rotators, since these two groups are commonly ignored by the patient, resulting in adhesive capsulitis or other disuse problems. In the case of the above-elbow amputee, the muscles about the shoulder all need emphasis, particularly the abductors and extensors. It is important in the above-elbow and higher-level amputee to educate and acquaint the patient with the movement known as biscapular abduction as early as possible. This motion is not commonly used by normal adults to perform any activity of daily living, and therefore most amputees find this motion difficult to learn at first. In addition, shoulder elevation and depression may also be introduced.

Compression Wrapping Although the upper-extremity amputation site is not a weight-bearing joint, there is a need to apply consistent compressive dressings to reduce volume and remove edema from the residual limb. This may be done using a compression bandage or stump shrinker. If a compression bandage is used it is best applied in a figure-8 fashion similar to that done for below-knee amputees. The keys to any compression wrap are to apply pressure more distally than proximally, to make oblique turns rather than circular turns, and to complete coverage of the limb as quickly as possible. In the shorter above-elbow amputations it may be necessary to incorporate some compression bandage around the other axilla to secure and suspend the wrap. It is important in the long below-elbow and the long above-elbow residual limbs not to choke the remaining extremity by circumferential pressure, creating a tourniquet. In the shoulder disarticulation or forequarter level, wrapping may serve primarily to hold surgical dressings in place rather than to promote any great amount of volume reduction.

Preparatory Prostheses. Preparatory prostheses in the upper extremity are perhaps more important than in the lower extremity, and certainly the timing of such prostheses is critical. In elective surgical cases, preparatory prostheses need to be discussed with amputees prior to amputation so that they understand the goals as well as the specific details of the hardware to be used. Studies by Malone et al,[1] Burkhalter et al,[14] and others indicate that there is a critical period of time following unilateral upper-extremity amputation in which preparatory prostheses must be fitted. If upper-extremity amputees are allowed to develop one-handed skills and are not fitted early with temporary or preparatory prostheses, the likelihood of those amputees wearing and using an upper-extremity prosthesis is very low. Malone et al[1] report on elective amputation done for brachial plexus injuries in which myoelectrically controlled prostheses were delivered quickly in a preparatory system allowing the client to quickly learn the control and use of the prosthesis. In nonelective upper extremity amputations, it is often difficult to fit early prostheses to patients with multiple skin flaps or staged procedures. However, it is still important that patients be fitted as soon as medically indicated with preparatory prostheses.

Preparatory prostheses may be made of plaster, plastic, or any of the newer plastics impregnated with resin, such as Cutter cast or Scotch cast. The length of these devices is not absolutely critical. Function is critical, and many others have eluded to the necessity for these devices to be functionally a part of the amputees early rehabilitation program. In addition to beginning the process of residual-limb maturation and exercise, temporary or preparatory prostheses may actually assist the amputee in activities of daily living such as feeding, dressing, or helping in the room while still in the hospital or at home following discharge.

To maximize the chances for a successful functional fitting of an upper-extremity prosthesis, a check socket may be used. Check sockets may be made of several materials. Included in this group are plaster, beeswax, clear plastic such as Surlyn, or low-temperature thermoplastics such as orthoplast or aquaplast. It is important that the prosthetist evaluate the height and position of the trim lines so that any compromise between range of motion, suspension, and function can be made and, more importantly, be understood by the amputee before the final delivery of the prosthesis. Once the check socket has been fitted and evaluated by both prosthetist and patient, a positive model is made from the check socket, and the definitive prosthesis is made from that positive model.

REFERENCES

1. Malone JH, Childers SJ, Underwood J, Leal JH. Immediate postsurgical management of upper-extremity amputation: Conventional, electric, and myoelectric prosthesis. *Orthot Prosthet*. 1981; **35**(2):1–9.

2. Kay HW, Newman JD. Relative incidence of new amputations. *Orthot Prosthet*. 1975; **29**(2):3–16.

3. Bender LF. *Prostheses and Rehabilitation After Arm Amputation*. Springfield, Ill: Charles C. Thomas; 1974.

4. Bunnell S. *Surgery of the Hand*. ed. 3. Philadelphia, Pa: Lippincott; 1956.

5. Tooms RE. Amputation surgery in the upper extremity. *Orthop Clin North Am*. 1972; 3(2):383–395.

6. Burkhalter WE, Hampton FL, Smeltzer JS. Wrist disarticulation and below-elbow amputation. In: Atlas of Limb Prosthetics, American Academy of Orthopaedic Surgeons. St. Louis, Mo: Mosby; 1981; 183–191.

7. Taylor C. The biomechanics of the normal and of the amputated upper extremity. In: Klopsteig PE, Wilson PD, eds. *Human Limbs and Their Substitutes*. New York: McGraw-Hill; 1954; 169–221.

8. Shurr DG, Cooper RR, Buckwalter JA, Blair WF. The terminal transverse congenital deficiency of the forearm. *Orthot Prosthet*. 1981; 3:22–25.

9. Sorbye R. Myoelectric prosthetic fitting in young children. *Clin Orthop*. 1980; **148**:34–40.

10. Hagg GM, Klasson B. Miniaturized electronic event counter. *Scand J Rehabil Med*. **60** (suppl) 6: 1978; 28–32.

11. Trost FJ. A comparison of conventional and myo-electric below-elbow prosthetic use. *Int Clin Info Bull*. 1983; **18**:9–16.

12. Northmore-Ball MD, Heger H, Hunter GA. The below-elbow myoelectric prostheses: A comparison of Otto Bock myoelectric prosthesis with the hook and functional hand. *J Bone Joint Surg*. 1980; **62B**(3):363–367.

13. Stein RB, Waller M. Functional comparison of upper extremity amputees using myoelectric and conventional prostheses. *Arch Phys Med Rehabil*. 1983; **64**:243–248.

14. Burkhalter WE, Mayfield G, Carmona LS. The upper-extremity amputee. *J Bone Joint Surg*. 1976; **58A**(1):46–51.

CHAPTER 9

Upper-Extremity Orthotics

This chapter will present a discussion of the etiology of problems requiring upper-extremity orthotics, a brief review of hand functions, and a discussion of orthotic components.

OVERVIEW OF UPPER-EXTREMITY ORTHOTICS

The hand is one part of the human anatomy that, more than any other, is treated by many health care professionals. Reasons for treatment by such a diverse group vary, perhaps even for well-intended philosophies. The hand may be cared for initially by a general practitioner, an orthopaedic surgeon, a hand surgeon, a plastic surgeon, a general surgeon, or a traumatologist or emergency room physician. Following the initial diagnosis and treatment plan, the patient may be cared for by a physical therapist, an occupational therapist, a hand therapist, a nurse, or an orthotist/prosthetist. Depending on the availability and organization, hand patients are cared for by a diverse group with equally diverse goals and philosophies. Whoever agrees to care for hand patients needs only two basic prerequisites: basic knowledge of hand anatomy, kinesiology, and care; and a desire to work closely with the managing physician or surgeon and patient.

ETIOLOGY

Problems leading to the use of hand orthoses can be categorized into three general groups: trauma, congenital problems, and reconstruction following disease.

Trauma
By far the most common patient etiology is the hand-trauma group. These injuries occur in all parts of life, from accidents, to work-related mishaps, to burns, to injuries associated with other injuries, such as Volkmann's ischemic contracture associated with the fracture of the humerus and subsequent severance of the brachial artery. Many hand-trauma cases also occur while working around the house.

Congenital Problems

Congenital hand defects come in a varied array of groups, including the syndactyly, or webbed fingers; central defects, where central or middle digits are absent; and polydactyly, or too many fingers. Larger hand-and-arm conditions include radial and ulnar club hand and brachydactyly, or short fingers, with concomitant dysplasia of the entire extremity.

Disease

The reconstructive patient may carry a variety of diagnoses, usually the destructive, collagen-vascular diseases like rheumatoid arthritis or lupus erythematosis. The patients often undergo numerous surgical procedures to reconstruct the deformed hand, bone, joints, soft tissue, tendons, or skin. Many postoperative situations call for the expertise of a therapist knowledgeable in the care of hands.

TYPES OF HAND SPLINTS

Splints connote many different things to caregivers, patients, and surgeons. The role of provision of such a splint may be shared, just as the care postinjury or postoperatively may be shared. Generally splints may occur in two forms, either temporary or definitive.

Temporary Versus Definitive Splints

Temporary splinting is often thought to be done for a primary purpose; may be altered upon change in condition; should be lightweight, strong, easily donned and doffed; should cost little or nothing; and should provide all biomechanical forces necessary to treat the pathology or need. Needless to say, few if any splints rate high in all categories.

From an orthotists' point of view, the time such a splint is needed must be established early, by the surgeon, in cooperation with therapists so that construction and materials may be consistent with goals. This will prevent situations in which a definitive splint is made for a problem only requiring temporary materials. Generally temporary splints may be constructed of plaster, fiberglass cast, low-temperature thermoplastics, or moldable sheet thermoplastics. Aluminum or steel are usually not considered temporary.

Static Versus Dynamic Splints

In addition to being temporary or definitive, hand splints are also designed to be static or dynamic. Generally speaking, static splints are thought to be resting, or positional, splints used to position or to hold a hand or wrist. Dynamic splints are splints that provide a dynamic force, generally using energy-storing materials like rubberbands, spring steel, wound, coiled wire, or plastic with memory. By the design of the splint, a portion of the hand is held or secured while the dynamic force is gently applied. Often this is done to reduce or "direct" the results of scar tissue.

Dynamic splints may direct forces at the small joints of the fingers, the wrist, or the entire hand and wrist. Due to the anatomy of the hand, advantage may be gained by prepositioning the wrist to attain the desired stretch of the finger. An example of this is the tenodesis effect. When the wrist extends, the fingers flex (metacarpophalangeal, MCP). This natural occurrence may be harnessed to provide useful motion and function.

HAND FUNCTIONS

There are four phases of hand function: reach, prehension, carry, and release. Reach requires good range of motion (ROM) in all joints, proximal stabilization, and muscle power in the extensor groups. Following reach, to get the hand to the mouth, 10 to 15 degrees of glenohumeral flexion is required. In the absence of flexion, more wrist flexion must be used.

Prehension may also be referred to as grip. Prehension patterns are primary functions of the hand. There are three main categories: pinch, grasp, and hook. Pinch may be tip, palmar, or lateral. Tip places the object between index finger tip and thumb, with the key to the definition including interphalangeal (IP) and distal interphalangeal (DIP) joint flexion. Tip pinch is usually used for smaller articles and often employs decreased strength. Palmar prehension, or three-jawed chuck, is the most commonly used form, accounting for 60% of all hand activities. This form uses the thumb, index, and long fingers, with the thumb pad placed directly under the fingers. It uses the median nerve, motor, and sensory distribution. Lateral prehension, or key grip, positions the thumb over the flexed proximal interphalangeal (PIP) joint of the index finger. It is called key grip because often keys are placed in locks in this fashion. Severe rheumatoid arthritics who have lost collateral structures of the MCP joints of index through small finger often use this grip. Normally, and in patients with rheumatoid arthritis (RA), key or lateral prehension generates more force than tip or palmer.

Tip, palmar, and lateral are prehensions used to manipulate objects to function during activities of daily living. Cylinder, spherical, and hook are gross grasps used to hold rather than to manipulate. Cylinder grasp fashions the hand around a cylinder with the MCP slightly flexed, the PIPs flexed to 75 degrees of flexion, and the thumb opposed under the index and long fingers. Spherical grip may be described as in holding a tennis ball, with the thumb slightly abducted and extended rather than opposed, as in cylinder grasp. Hook grip is often thought of as the "link grip," linking ape prehension with human and using all fingers, particularly the PIP joints, without using the thumb.

Often students new to the anatomy and kinesiology of the hand confuse thumb extension and abduction. Abduction of the thumb carpometacarpal (CMC) joints involves motion away from the plane of the palm, usually including partial opposition, at least under the index and long pads, as in palmar prehension. Thumb extension of the CMC joint involves motion in the plane of the palm. Note that extension of the thumb IP joint may occur with the thumb CMC joint either abducted/opposed or extended.

Conditions Affecting the Use of Hand Splints

Any therapist or orthotist working in the area of hand care should be acquainted with the basic science involved in stiffness and scarring associated with edema. Many sources are available. One recent resource of note is *Hand Rehabilitation*,[1] in the *Clinics in Physical Therapy* series, edited very aptly by Christine A. Moran, RPT.

The physiology of scar formation is important in hand care. Following injury, surgery, or infection in the hand, protein-rich exudate invades the narrow passages between layers of tissue in the hand. Since the body uses fibroblasts to seal off infection, normal blood does not carry away the fibroblasts. If the tissue planes do not move, either due to pain, surgical implants, edema, or hand splints, fibrosis occurs very early on. Thus, although hand splints may assist hand care by preventing unwanted motion, this goal must be carefully considered along with the concomitant outcome of stiffness via protein-rich exudate and immobilization.

A.E. Flatt (personal communication, 1978) believes that scar formation and remodeling occurs from day 1 through 18 months postinjury. He states that scar formation is always present following the 18-month period, with the amount and severity of loss of motion and function determined by genetics of patient, type and severity of injury, number of surgical procedures in relatively short period of time, postoperative care, therapist/patient cooperation, and appropriate orthotic management.

Hardy[1] quotes Weber and Davis in her chapter on scar formation: "Hand therapy is behavioral modification of the fibroblast during the healing response."[1] (p 8) Gribben[2] (p 170), in her chapter on splinting raises nine questions essential to be answered before splinting any patient:

1. Identification of primary, secondary, and associated problems?
2. What do I expect to accomplish through the use of a splint?
3. What splint components are integral to correction of the problems?
4. What splint design will best encompass these components?
5. Should the splint be static or dynamic?
6. Should the base be volar or dorsal?
7. What joints should be included in the splint?
8. What is the patient's level of cognition? Is it adequate for correct wearing, and usage of the splint?
9. What is the patient's emotional status?

Once a decision to splint has been agreed upon by all team members (including the patient), a design must emerge. So-called off-the-shelf splints are denounced by many and used by most. However, off-the-shelf or noncustom devices of all kinds suffer from the old adage of "fitting everyone, and therefore no one." Fortunately there is some middle ground, as many patients may be successfully custom fitted using readily available and premade orthoses.

There are many who believe custom-made orthoses are necessary for each and every patient. In such cases impressions made from plaster or alginate may be used as well as patterns formed and orthoses constructed. Obviously the very large and very small and one-of-a-kind cases require custom design as well as construction. The ultimate answer to custom *v* custom-fitted hand orthoses rests with the skill and clientele of the therapist, the numbers of support staff available, and/or the availability of an interested and knowledgeable orthotist.

UPPER-EXTREMITY ORTHOTIC COMPONENTS

The best complete system of hand orthoses available in America today is the Mannerfelt system, developed by Lutz Biedermann, CPO, of West Germany. It is available in three sizes of rights and lefts. Consistent with lower-limb orthotics and prosthetics, the Mannerfelt system is modular, allowing all components to be added as needed or removed if unnecessary.

Examples of Splinting Systems

Figure 9–1 demonstrates one version of a long opponens. The long opponens contains at least a short-opponens hand piece and a wrist/forearm component, either attached solidly or with a spring tension to produce wrist dorsiflexion. Another version of the wrist joint produces spring-assisted ulnar deviation, used for rheumatoid arthritics.

Figure 9–2 demonstrates the short-opponens splint, which acts to support the arches of the metacarpals, both transversely and longitudinally. In addition, it may position the thumb CMC and MP or IP joints and prevents contracture of or stretches the thumb-index web space. This is also referred to as a thumb-adduction stop. Lastly, the short opponens provides a point from which more distal components may attach.

Figure 9–3 demonstrates the dynamic finger-extension assist. This component is used when finger joint MPs are stiff or when radial nerve injury renders extension difficult or impossible. Since finger flexors still function, patients are able to hold light objects without active extensors. When stiff PIP finger joints affect finger MCP joint motion (hyperextension), a lumbrical bar or MP extension stop may be added. Figure 9–4 shows the stop in place, using PIP assists and long-opponens splint.

Figure 9–5 demonstrates a long opponens, with dynamic wrist-extension assist. This may be used when wrist-flexion contracture exists, when only wrist extension is

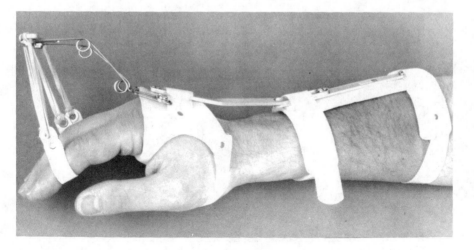

Figure 9–1. A long opponens wrist-hand orthosis. (From Becker Orthopaedic, with permission.)

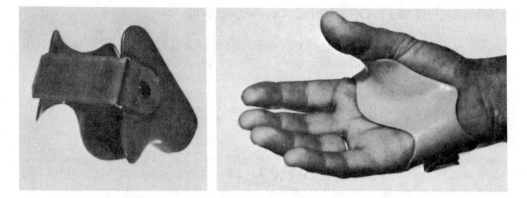

Figure 9–2. A short opponens.

interrupted (neurologically), or following scarring to the volar wrist crease, when passive wrist extension is limited.

Figure 9–4 demonstrates the dynamic wrist long opponens, PIP extension assist with lumbrical bar or MP extension stop. These are often used following major trauma to the volar wrist, when tendons, nerves, and bone may be cut or crushed. Thus in addition to skin and joint tightness or contracture, flexor tendon and nerves may also be scarred following surgical repair.

Figure 9–6 demonstrates the dynamic application of forces to produce increased flexion of finger joints used following injury to the extensor or dorsal part of the hand. Gently dynamic force over time will produce increased joint motion.

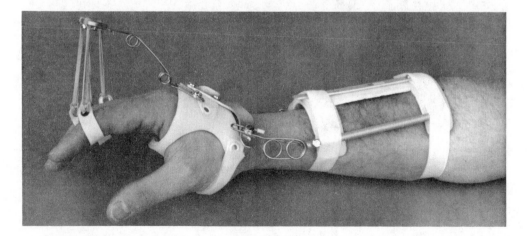

Figure 9–3. A spring-wrist extension assist with MCP extension assist. (From Becker Orthopaedic, with permission.)

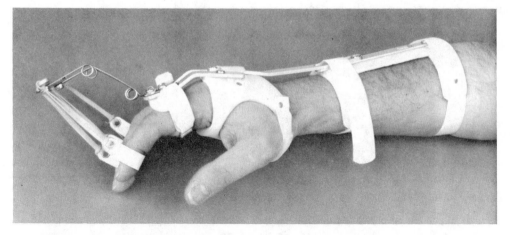

Figure 9–4. A dynamic long opponens, PIP extension assist with lumbrical bar or MCP extension stop. (From Becker Orthopaedic, with permission.)

Externally Powered Upper-Extremity Orthoses. Since the development of the McKibben muscle, a CO_2-filled latex rubber bladder, orthotists and therapists have attempted to provide externally powered upper-extremity orthotic systems to cervical spine-injured clients. Problems with air tanks and latex rubber bladders have given way to electric motors, but the problems of "gadget tolerance" or intolerance remain.

Beard and Long[3] followed usage of externally powered devices for over 12 years, concluding that only one third indicated that they used their device following discharge from the rehabilitation center. They cite the following problems[3](p 2):

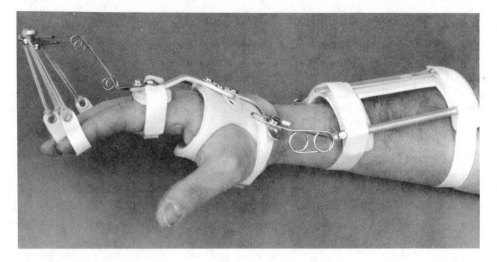

Figure 9–5. A long opponens with dynamic wrist-extension assist. (From Becker Orthopaedic, with permission.)

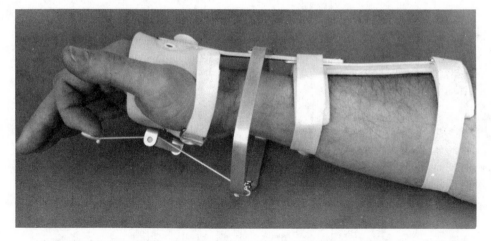

Figure 9–6. MCP and PIP flexion assist. (From Becker Orthopaedic, with permission.)

poor quality of performance and the small number of activities which can be accomplished, due to limited range of motion and lack of forceful movement, lead to disuse. Without good proximal arm function, the externally powered hand splint is apparently of little value to these patients. The additional time required for application of the entire system is not justified. Poor quality of performance of activities was the reason most frequently cited by patients for disuse of externally-powered orthoses.

Because of the aforementioned problems, Hoy and Guilford[4] developed the functional ratchet system. This system, attached to a reciprocating wrist orthosis, or tenodesis splint, allows palmar prehension via wrist extension. The adjustable, spring-loaded ratchet maintains prehension of the object until the ratchet is released, at which time the wrist flexes and the hand releases the object.

State of the Art in Upper-Extremity Orthotics
From 1975 through 1985, 21 articles about orthotics and the upper extremity appeared in *Orthotics and Prosthetics*, the official publication of the American Association of Orthotists and Prosthetists. Of these articles none developed criteria from which clinical trials could be compared.

Crochetiere et al[5] mentioned that 11 Granger orthoses had been fitted. However, no patient data were reported, and no comparisons were made with any other orthoses nor reports of functional tests given. Katz et al[6] presented a case report providing a standard voluntary-opening terminal device for a C-6 quadriplegic. The report mentioned using functional tasks. No comparisons were made with other devices or with the absence of a device.

The fact that only two of 21 articles presented any clinical data demonstrates the lack of clinical interest in orthoses of the upper extremity. Twenty-one articles in 10 years also indicates less than enthusiasm about the upper extremity. The lack of good clinical usefulness and relevance of orthoses for the upper extremity leads one to question the true contribution to the field made by upper-extremity orthoses. It also must make one question the time spent on both the academics and the certification process of becoming a certified orthotist.

REFERENCES

1. Hardy MA. Preserving Function in the Inflamed and Acutely Injured Hand. In: Moran C, ed. *Hand Rehabilitation. New York, NY: Churchill Livingston; 1986.*
2. Gribben M. Splinting principles for hand injuries. In: Moran C, ed. *Hand Rehabilitation.* New York, NY: Churchill Livingston; 1986.
3. Beard JE, Long C. Follow-up study on usage of externally-powered orthoses. *Orthot Prosthet.* 1970; **24**(2):2.
4. Hoy DJ, Guilford AW. The functional ratchet orthotic system. *Orthot Prosthet.* 1978; **32**(2):21–24.
5. Crochetiere W, Goldstein S, Granger CV, Ireland J. The "Granger" orthosis for radial nerve palsy. *Orthot Prosthet.* 1975; **29**(4):27–31.
6. Katz JA, et al. A case study: Use of a terminal device to augment a paralyzed hand. *Orthot Prosthet.* 1983; **37**(4):49–53.

CHAPTER 10

Juvenile Amputees

This chapter discusses juvenile, including congenital, amputees. As was the case with hip disarticulation amputation, juvenile amputees are not commonly encountered in a typical general hospital setting; but they do represent unique challenges. This chapter presents an overview of factors to consider when dealing with these special individuals.

THE JUVENILE AMPUTEE

Before discussing the juvenile amputee, several people must be mentioned for their outstanding work in this area. The works of these authors are essential reading for anyone whose clinical practice includes work with a large number of children. Physicians include George Aitken, Claude Lambert, Lawrence Friedman, Robert Tooms, Leon Kruger, and Y. Setoguchi. Prosthetists of note include Ronnie Snell, CP; Carman Tablada, CP; Bert Titus, CPO; and C. Corriveau, CPO. Therapists of note include Jeannette Hutchison, PT/OT; Ruth Rosenfelder, RPT; Julie Shaperman, OTR; and Helen Vaughn, RPT. Many of these professionals have cared for juvenile amputees in area centers around the United States for over 30 years. Their collective work is what we know today as childrens' prosthetics.

Etiology

Aitken[1] defined the juvenile amputee as a skeletally immature person with an amputation or congenital limb deficiency. As director of the Grand Rapids, MI, Area Amputee Project for many years, Aitken reported that juvenile upper-extremity amputations are more often congenital than acquired due to trauma, disease, or tumor.

Congenital Amputation. Congenital means present at birth and may be either a limb deficiency, due to underdevelopment of a limb segment, or a true congenital amputation, where the distal part was once present but was severed sometime before birth. (These differences, although subtle, will become more important as further classifications emerge later in this chapter.) In Aitken's[1] study, 372 of 1,210 (30.7%) patients who had true congenital amputations had two or more affected limbs. One hundred eleven of the 372 congenital amputees were affected in all four limbs. Although Aitken's[1] group may represent a skewed sample, the fact remains that congenital limb deficiency often affects multiple limbs (Fig. 10–1).

Acquired Amputation. In Aitken's[1] study, 850 of 923 (92%) acquired amputations affected only one limb. Aitken's[1] data indicated that vehicular accidents led the list of causes for acquired amputations. The next three most common causes were power tools (farm machinery), gunshot/explosion injuries, and railroad injuries. Together these four causes accounted for 75% of acquired amputations in children.

Disease-Related Amputation. Tumor is the largest single cause of disease-related amputation in children. Other reasons might include vascular compromise, often in the form of thrombi secondary to disease, and other miscellaneous etiologies.

Surgical Conversion. The concept of surgical conversion involves a surgical "correction" to change an existing anatomic entity into one that can be more realistically fitted with a functional prosthesis. A common example is an ankle disarticulation procedure that is done in the case of a poorly developed or contractured foot. In this example the foot is surgically converted into a more usable residual limb, one that can be more easily and cosmetically fitted with standard prosthetic components.

Aitken reported that 50.8% of lower-extremity congenital-limb deficiencies required surgical conversion, while only 7.9% of upper-limb deficiencies required sur-

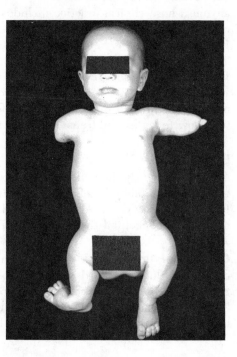

Figure 10–1. Congenital quadramembral amputee. (From Shurr DG, Cooper RR, Buckwalter JA, Blair WF. Juvenile amputees classification and revision rates. *Orthot Prosthet.* 1982; **36**:24, with permission)

gery. Often upper-limb anatomic segments can provide adequate function despite the presence of unusual anatomic configurations. Additionally, intact anatomic segments provide sensibility, something modern prosthetics can, as yet, not do.

The Young Amputee

The juvenile amputee is *not* simply a miniature version of an adult amputee. Likewise, juvenile amputees are not fitted with components that were designed for adults and miniaturized for children. The juvenile amputee is a growing person whose residual limb, especially its length, is always changing. The juvenile amputee is continually dependent on parents, society, and the prosthetic clinic team, since growth spurts can render a prosthesis too small and/or too short in a matter of weeks. The juvenile is malleable both physically and emotionally, often making certain aspects of treatment easier than with some adults. Since the physical body is malleable, the requirements of strict socket fit are more relaxed, making it possible to extend the normal useful life of a prosthesis. Rarely do juvenile amputees complain of pain or develop stump ulcers, and most can tolerate rubbing and skin irritation that might cause a serious problem for an older dysvascular amputee.

Emotionally juveniles adapt readily to various situations, allowing prosthetic fitting and gait training to occur with few complications. As compared to adults, children can often be walking independently with a prosthesis in a few days, whereas many adults may require more training.

Availability and Delivery of Services. Juveniles, like some adults, are not highly educated or self-supporting. Many states have Crippled Childrens Clinics and various privately sponsored childrens clinics that provide prosthetic care. Additionally, Variety Clubs nationwide provide a great deal of support for upper-extremity prostheses for children. The Shriners hospitals all over America provide general orthopaedic care, which includes prosthetic care, to many juveniles free of charge. Unfortunately children seeking care from these specialized centers often need to travel great distances and are not cared for locally. For these reasons the care of the juvenile amputee may present special problems for the physical therapist, prosthetist, and surgeon. Optimal surgical treatment and prosthetic fitting require careful planning and frequent clinical and radiographic follow-up, as growth alters the size and configuration of the residual limb.

Growth. To anticipate the eventual growth of the long bones, the relative contribution of the epiphyses is important. In the lower extremity, 70% of the length of the femur depends on the distal femoral epiphysis, while about 60% of the tibia and fibula come from the proximal epiphyses. Therefore the epiphyses around the knee contribute 67% to the overall length of the lower limb. In the upper extremity, 80% of the length originates from the proximal epiphysis, whereas the distal epiphyses of the radius and ulna provide overall growth to the arm and forearm. Loss or absence of these epiphyses may alter the eventual length of the limb, resulting in significant limb-length discrepancies.

The Problem of Bony Overgrowth. In juvenile amputees, growth of the bones of the residual limb and the soft tissues may be disproportionate, resulting in bony overgrowth. This problem, as stated by Lambert,[2] represents the most common unfavorable sequela of the surgical treatment of the juvenile amputee. Aitken,[3] Lambert,[2] and Pellicore[4] describe the bony overgrowth in the juvenile amputee as appositional bone growth independent of epiphyseal growth. Aitken[5] reported the order of overgrowth frequency as humerus, fibula, tibia, femur, and tibia/fibula. Once the bone pierces the skin, treatment usually includes bony excision and soft-tissue closure. Pellicore[4] demonstrated that in addition to the specific bone involved, age at amputation and occurrence of transection through bone influence the recurrence of bony overgrowth. According to him, the bones involved, in order of frequency were tibia, humerus, fibula, femur, and tibia/fibula. He and Aitken[1] concluded that prevention of overgrowth can best be accomplished by joint disarticulation.

Classification of Juvenile Amputees

Parents of juvenile amputees often request information from medical personnel concerning the anticipated nature and frequency of surgical and prosthetic modification that may be necessary due to bony overgrowth. Ideally classification of the juvenile amputee by type, age and bones involved, and an analysis of patients with such classifications should help to answer these questions.

Many children with acquired amputations need revision, particularly of the humerus and fibula (Fig. 10–2). True congenital amputations that need revision, although

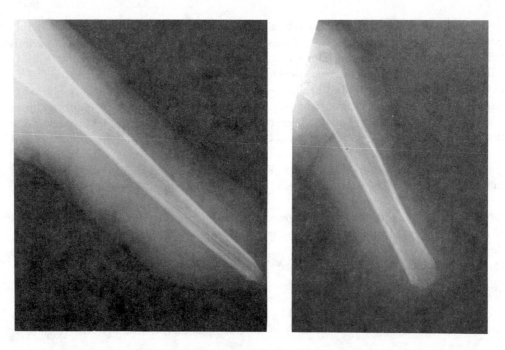

Figure 10–2. Bony overgrowth of the humerus, before, on left, and after surgical revision. (From Shurr DG, Cooper RR, Buckwalter JA, Blair WF. Juvenile amputees classification and revision rates. *Orthot Prosthet.* 1982; **36**:23, with permission.)

rare, were reported by Lambert[2] and Aitken and Franz[6] but were not described in detail. Shurr et al[6] reviewed 120 patients with major limb deficiencies or amputations prior to skeletal maturity and developed a five-part classification scheme (Table 10–1).

Type I cases included acquired amputations. The amputees in this group ranged from 3 months to 14 years of age at the time of amputation. Seven cases were skeletally mature. The humerus was found to show bony overgrowth most frequently and required as many as six surgical revisions, demanding a total of 14 procedures on four of the patients. The fibula was revised in three cases, the tibia/fibula twice, and the tibia alone once. Only one of these occurred at the above-elbow level, and only one case required separate revisions of the tibia and fibula on an amputation that had been acquired at the age of 10 years. These revisions were done at the ages of 15 and 16 years, respectively. Individuals acquiring an amputation after the age of 12 years needed no revision, regardless of the bone involved.

Type II cases, true congenital amputations, are defined as amputations through the long bones that are present at birth. Shurr et al[7] excluded from this type the classical terminal-transverse below-elbow deficiency with vestigial hand or nubbins and all other congenital limb deficiencies not through the long bones. This latter group (phocomelias and amelias, PFFD) are included in type V. The distinction between type II and type V amputations is important. Type II includes only true congenital amputations through long bone and may result from defects such as constriction-ring syndromes.

Of the eight type II cases reviewed, seven underwent at least one revision. One fibula was revised five times, and two humeri were revised twice. Of interest was one patient (Fig. 10–1) who had bilateral PFFD and bilateral above-elbow amputations, one longer than the other. In 20 years he had undergone two revisions for the right side and no revisions for the left side. Type II congenital, through-bone amputations were found to overgrow. The humerus, the bone involved most often, required six revisions in four patients. Two tibia/fibulae were revised a total of four times: three in one case and one in another (Table 10–2). Since all patients in type II had at least three limbs involved and had at least simple syndactylys, this group appears to respond differently than the classical limb-deficient patient with only one limb involved. From the data, patients with congenital amputations of the humerus and fibula react much like type I or type III, even though they appear to be true congenital amputees.

TABLE 10-1. CLASSIFICATION OF JUVENILE AMPUTATIONS

Type	Description	Number of Cases
I	Acquired amputations (infection, trauma, etc)	26
II	Congenital amputations through long bones	8
III	Congenital deficiencies surgically converted by amputation through bone	3
IV	Congenital deficiencies surgically converted by disarticulation	4
V	Congenital deficiencies treated nonsurgically with prostheses	79
		120

From Shurr D. G., Cooper, R. R., Buckwalter, J. A., Blair, W. F., Juvenile amputees: Classification and revision rates. Orthot Prosthet. 1981; **36**:24, with permission.

TABLE 10-2. TYPE II CONGENITAL AMPUTATIONS THROUGH THE LONG BONES

Level	Follow-up (Years)	Number of Revisions	Age (Years) at Revision		
			Humerus	*Fibula*	*Tibia/Fibula*
AE	8	1	7		
AE	8	2	8, 10		
AE	3	1	2		
BK	14	3			2, 4, 14
(L)AE	20		3, 7		
(R)AE		2(R)			
BK	7	1			5
BK	9	5		1, 3, 6, 7, 9	

Note: AE = above elbow; BK = below knee.
*From Shurr D. G., Cooper, R. R., Buckwalter, J. A., Blair, W. F. Juvenile amputees Classification and revision rates. Orthot Prosthet. 1981; **36**:27, with permission.*

Type III cases are those in which surgical conversion of congenital limb deficiency required cutting through a long bone. In the group studied by Shurr et al,[7] all were at the below-knee level. Two were congenital pseudarthroses of the tibia and fibula, and one was a congenital absence of the fibula. Like the type I amputations, type III required surgical revision. Of the below-knee amputees, two needed revision of the tibia, one at the age of 12 years and one at the age of 15 years, and one required revision of the fibula. All amputations had been done prior to the age of 5 years and predictably acted similarly to type I amputations.

Type IV encompasses congenital deficiencies converted surgically by disarticulation. PFFD and single- or double-ray feet without a hindfoot are examples. Surgical conversion in this group usually enhanced prosthetic fitting without concomitant loss in function. No bony overgrowth occurred in this group.

Type V, making up the largest subgroup of congenital deficiencies treated non-surgically, includes the classical terminal-transverse below-elbow amputation that occurs more often in females and on the left side (Table 10–3). A vestigial hand or nubbins are usually present. In a review of 33 unilateral cases with no other abnormalities, no cases of bony overgrowth were found.

After reviewing this group of juvenile amputees, Shurr et al[7] concluded that the above-described classification system is valuable for prognostic purposes. The known tendency of acquired amputations (type I) to require revision, sometimes multiple revisions, was confirmed. Twenty-six patients underwent 21 revisions. The younger the patient at the time of amputation, the more likely the need for revision. The humerus was most often revised, followed by the fibula, tibia/fibula, and tibia. The analysis indicated that congenital transverse amputations (type II) through long bones frequently require revision, occurring 14 times in seven patients and thus confirming the opinions of Aitken[6] and Lambert.[2] For prognostic purposes, the transverse congenital amputation (type II) should be considered an entity distinctly different from non-surgically treated congenital terminal-transverse deficiencies (type V) in which revisions were not required.

TABLE 10-3. OCCURRENCE OF CONGENITAL BELOW-ELBOW AMPUTATIONS

	Shurr[10] (1980)	Birch-Jensen[8] (1949)	Aitken and Frantz[6] (1955)	Aitken and O'Rahilly[9] (1961)
Total number of patients studied	48	161	49	331
Male	19 (40%)	69 (43%)	22 (45%)	156 (47%)
Female	29 (60%)	92 (57%)	27 (55%)	175 (53%)
Left	35 (69%)	108 (67%)	37 (76%)	212 (64%)
Right	16 (31%)	53 (33%)	12 (24%)	119 (36%)

From Shurr, DG., Cooper, RR., Buckwalter, JA., Blair, W.F. Terminal transverse congenital limb deficiency of the forearm. Orthot Prosthet. 1981; 35:23, with permission.

When congenital deficiencies were treated by amputation through long bones (type III), they behaved, relative to surgical revision, as a congenital amputation through long bone. The congenital deficiency treated by amputation through long bone changed from an entity in which revision was unlikely to one in which revision was nearly predictable. If the congenital deficiency was surgically treated by disarticulation instead of amputation (type IV), revision was not necessary, reaffirming that, when possible, disarticulation is the preferred surgical procedure.

Terminal-Transverse Congenital Limb Deficiency of the Forearm

Birch-Jensen[8] examined the records of over 4 million patients to determine the incidence of this common below-elbow limb deficiency. In this classic study (Table 10–3) 161 patients were identified as congenital below-elbow amputees, 69 male and 92 female. A total of 108 occurred on the left, and 53 occurred on the right side. Aitken and Franz[6] reported a total of 49 patients; 22 males and 27 females, 37 left sided and 12 right sided. In a series published by Aitken and O'Rahilly,[9] a total of 331 cases were reviewed. Of these, 156 were male, 175 female; 212 were left sided and 119 were right sided. Shurr[10] identified 48 patients with this below-elbow amputation. These patients were placed into two groups: group 1 having unilateral below-elbow congenital amputation and group 2 patients with associated anomalies, including four bilateral upper-extremity amputees. There were 19 males and 29 females. To complete the series one patient with a below-elbow amputation also had a contralateral elbow disarticulation, making a total of 52 amputations. Of 51 below-elbow amputations, 35 were on the left and 16 were on the right. The data in each of these studies agree with regard to relative incidence, indicating a predominance of females and a left-to-right ratio of nearly 2:1. The congenital below-elbow terminal-transverse amputation appears to be a distinct entity, well defined in its unilateral presentation. Early, aggressive fitting of prostheses at about 6 months of age, as described below, is well accepted by both parents and children.

Prosthetic Management of Juvenile Amputees

Timing of Prosthetic Fitting. The timing of fitting of artificial limbs should coincide with normal growth and development whenever possible. It becomes quite frustrating for both parents and amputee when progress is such that parents and patient fail to see the usefulness of the prosthesis. Juvenile amputees should not be expected to perform physical tasks any sooner than the normal developmental sequence allows. Therefore the prosthetic team members should be aware of certain developmental milestones and be able to relate these to the devices provided to the juvenile amputee.

The fitting of the lower extremity is often easy to time properly, since most parents are very aware of when children are expected to be able to walk. Prosthetic fitting of the lower-extremity juvenile amputee should be timed to coincide with standing, cruising, and eventually walking. Most experts agree that many babies sit alone at 6 months, pull to stand and cruise around furniture between 8 and 12 months, and walk independently between 12 and 15 months of age. Leg prostheses should be fitted in anticipation of these milestones.

The timing of the fitting of an upper-extremity prosthesis occurs often a bit earlier than the lower. The critical element in the upper extremity is to provide a device at the appropriate time that will allow the amputee to bring the hands together for bimanual hand activities (eg, patty cake). This type of prosthetic device will also provide two even-length arms with which to begin quadripedal crawling. Such an arm is often equipped with only a passive mitten hand with no cable and no moving parts (Fig. 10–3).

Parents need to be instructed with regard to evaluation of proper fit, means of donning and doffing, how to assist the child in using the device, what to expect functionally, and how to check the skin for signs of an ill-fitting prosthesis or tight harness. Ideally unilateral amputees should wear their prostheses all day beginning at a very early age. Regular return visits need to be scheduled to follow the child and to answer parents' questions.

Recently a number of prosthetic teams have begun fitting small children, less than 1 year of age, with myoelectrically controlled hands with grasped release. This appears to be contrary to evidence that shows that meaningful release does not normally appear until between the ages of 2 and 2½ years. Data from these fittings will either support or refute this concept in the near future.

When the child outgrows the initial prosthesis, usually at the age of 1½ to 2 years, a new socket is made, and a split-hook terminal device is introduced (Fig. 10–4). Care must be taken to educate the parents to the body motions needed to power the voluntary-opening terminal device. The timing of the first split-hook prosthesis allows about one year for the family to become accustomed to the child's amputation and to overcome the negative attitudes commonly associated with the use of a prosthetic hook, even though it may be clearly more functional than a prosthetic hand.

Voluntary-opening, body-powered hands are fitted at about the age of four years, since very few small hands are available in body-powered systems. Children's hooks sized 12 and 10 function from ages 2 to 9 years. At the age of 10 years the 9-series hooks are appropriate in terms of both size and desirability.

Prosthetic Wearers and Prosthetic Users. A successful wearer may be defined as a person who wears the prosthesis most of his or her waking hours. Using this definition,

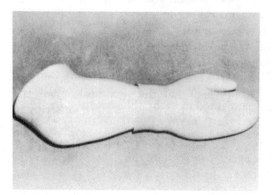

Figure 10–3. Below-elbow level first fitting with passive mitten. (From Shurr DG, Cooper RR, Buckwalter JA, Blair WF. Terminal transverse congenital limb deficiency of the forearm. *Orthot Prosthet.* 1981; **35**:23, with permission.)

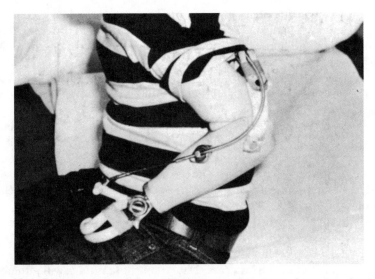

Figure 10–4. Below-elbow level fitting with split-hook TD. (From Shurr DG, Cooper RR, Buckwalter JA, Blair WF. Terminal transverse congenital limb deficiency of the forearm. Orthot Prosthet. 1981; **35**:24, with permission)

many successful wearers are fitted before the age of 1 year. It has been reported that parents of successful wearers express satisfaction with an aggressive, early-fitting approach. Parents also report that functional milestones are often delayed, including dressing independence and tying one's shoes. Most parents comment about the improved function of their child with the use of the prosthetic device. This is difficult to measure objectively, since no controls exist and since a comparison with a normal limb would be unfair. However, successful wearers are not necessarily successful users, and a successful user may not always be a successful wearer. Concerning the appearance of the prosthesis, parents often describe it as "cold," "clunky," "ugly," or "noisy"; but most of these same families admit that their child looks "naked without it."

Questions concerning deficiencies in the prosthetic device or hook indicate that most successful wearers and their families feel the devices are adequate. Many refer to the day in the future when a prosthetic hand will be as practical and useful as a hook. In contrast, many teenage children, who frequently are concerned about their appearance, report discontinuing use of a prosthesis between the ages of 13 to 20 years, only to return to prosthetic use at a later age. Others feel that the prosthesis gives the appearance of a "handicapped person," and going without anything is more satisfying to their self-image.

An unsuccessful wearer seldom wears the prosthesis. Unsuccessful wearers can be categorized as those who were fitted after the age of 5 years, and some after the age of 10 years. Drastic changes in wearing history appear to be rare.

REFERENCES

1. Aitken GT. *Course in Juvenile Amputation.* Northwestern University School of Medicine, 1976
2. Lambert CT. Amputation surgery in the child. *Orthop Clin North Am.* 1972; 3(2):476.
3. Aitken GT. Overgrowth of the amputation stump. *Int Clin Info Bull.* 1962; 1(11):1–8.
4. Pellicore RJ. Incidence of bone overgrowth in the juvenile amputee population. *Int Clin Info Bull.* 1974; 13(15):1–10.
5. Aitken GT. The child amputee. *Clin Orthop.* 1972; 3(2):476.
6. Aitken GT, Franz CH. Congenital amputation of the forearm. *Ann Surg.* 1955; 141:519–522.
7. Shurr DG, Cooper RR, Buckwalter J, Blair WB. Juvenile amputation: Classification and revision rates. *Orthot Prosthet.* 1982; 36(2):23–28.
8. Birch-Jensen A. *Congenital Deformities of the Upper Extremity.* Commission: Andelsbogtrykkeriet i Odense und det danske forlag; 1949. Thesis.
9. Aitken GT, O'Rahilly R. Congenital skeletal limb deficiencies. The area child amputee program. Michigan Crippled Children Program. Presented at Northwestern University Prosthetic-Orthotic Center; 1972; Chicago, Ill.
10. Shurr DG. Terminal transverse congenital limb deficiency of the forearm. *Orthot Prosthet.* 1981; 35(3):22–25.

CHAPTER 11

Spinal Orthotics

T his chapter will present a brief historical perspective on spinal orthotics, a consideration of the intended functions of spinal orthoses, the components of spinal orthoses, commonly prescribed spinal orthotic configurations, and clinical studies supporting their effects and effectiveness in the overall treatment of spinal disorders.

HISTORICAL PERSPECTIVE

The history of spinal orthotics may be traced to the ancient Greeks and Egyptians. Early records indicate that these cultures used tree bark that was cut circumferentially from the tree and then placed around the body of the patient with a spinal deformity or problem (Fig. 11–1). The configuration of the bark resembles very much the design and purpose of modern spinal orthoses that utilize metal, fabric, and plastic contoured to normal or abnormal spinal anatomy to produce the desired function. Today plastics of many kinds are replacing metal in spinal orthoses. Lightweight and washable plastics are easily molded, are usually remoldable, and offer the patient a cosmetic and comfortable orthosis.

FUNCTIONS OF SPINAL ORTHOSES

Lucas and Bresler[1] in 1961 described the spine as a modified elastic rod. When the base was fixed with only the intrinsic or ligamentous components in place, the largest load it could withstand without buckling was 2 kg. Clearly the extrinsic musculature plays a very important part in the overall stability of the human spine. In cases where the intrinsic structures are inadequate, a spinal orthosis may be required to provide extrinsic stability.

Clinical reasons for the use of spinal orthotics include immobilization, support, and correction/prevention of deformity. Immobilization orthoses are classically used for a large group of conditions, including trauma with or without surgical fixation or reconstruction. During this time there is a need to limit motion of portions of the spinal

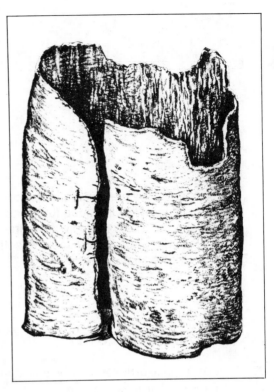

Figure 11–1. Ancient tree-bark spinal orthosis.

column. Since spinal orthoses may be worn for a period of weeks or months, the material chosen and the fit are particularly important to both patient compliance and comfort.

Supportive orthoses may be thought of as those that provide temporary care in cases of pain in the cervical or thoracolumbar region of the spine. Principles employed in supportive orthoses are an increase in intra-abdominal pressure, a kinesthetic reminder or restraint of painful range of motion, and the application of pressure over the largest possible surface area. Cervical orthoses are almost always supportive or immobilizing, since most pathologies yield instability and not deformity of the cervical spine. Such supportive orthoses may be custom fabricated or prefabricated and custom fitted to each patient. Their successful use depends on choice of the appropriate orthosis following a complete diagnostic workup and professional custom fitting. Corrective orthoses include a large group of devices used primarily in growing children and for spinal diseases such as scoliosis and kyphosis.

COMPONENTS OF SPINAL ORTHOTICS

There are many components of spinal orthoses that are common to different devices, although the devices may have different designs and functions.

Thoracic Band

The most proximal component of any lumbosacral orthosis (LSO) or thoracic lumbosacral orthosis (TLSO) is the thoracic band (Fig. 11–2). The superior border of this component is 1 in inferior to the more inferior angle of the scapula. The lateral borders of the thoracic band are the midaxillary trochanteric lines (MATLs). The thoracic band allows attachment for other components, including the lateral uprights, the paraspinal uprights, or shoulder straps.

Pelvic Band

The pelvic band usually represents the most distal component of a spinal orthosis (Fig. 11–3). It lies inferiorly at the level of the sacrocoxygeal junction. Laterally the pelvic band extends to the MATL at the level between the greater trochanter and the iliac crest. In order for the pelvic band to be fitted properly, the contours over the buttocks should flow into the concavity of the gluteus maximus, allowing proper end support. This also gives rise to other components, such as the paraspinal uprights, the lateral uprights, and the apron or corset.

Paraspinal Uprights

Paraspinal uprights, or bars, are positioned parallel to the spine, being careful not to touch the transverse processes of the vertebrae (Fig. 11–4). They are bounded on the superior end by the thoracic band and on the inferior end by the pelvic band. These paraspinal bars may either be contoured to the lumbar lordosis or bridged to encourage lumbar spine flexion.

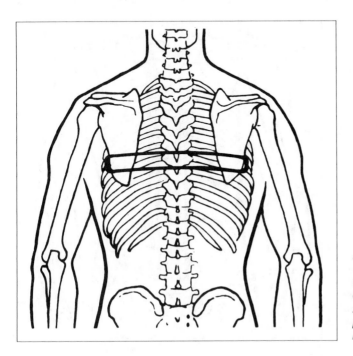

Figure 11–2. Thoracic band. (Reproduced by permission from Berger, N, Lusskin, R. Orthotic components and systems. In: *American Academy of Orthopaedic Surgeons: Atlas of Orthotics.* St. Louis, Mo: Mosby; 1975:)

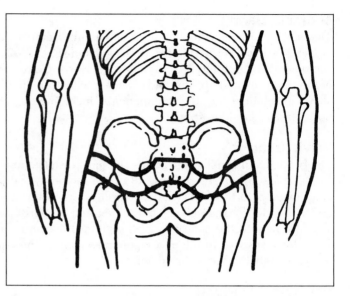

Figure 11–3. Pelvic band. (Reproduced by permission from Berger, N. Lusskin, R. Orthotic components and systems. In: *American Academy of Orthopaedic Surgeons: Atlas of Orthotics*. St. Louis, Mo: Mosby; 1975.)

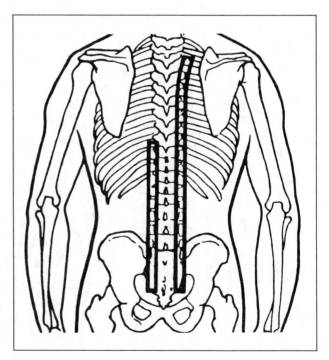

Figure 11–4. Paraspinal uprights or bars. (Reproduced by permission from Berger, N, Lusskin, R. Orthotic components and systems. In: *American Academy of Orthopaedic Surgeons: Atlas of Orthotics*. St. Louis, Mo: Mosby; 1975.)

Lateral Uprights

Lateral uprights, or bars, follow the MATL and connect the pelvic band and the thoracic band (Fig. 11–5). The lateral uprights connect the posterior half and the anterior half, providing attachment points for the apron or abdominal support.

Abdominal Support or Apron

The abdominal apron, or corset, makes up the anterior portion of many orthoses (Fig. 11–6). It lies superiorly 12 mm inferior to the xyphoid process of the sternum and inferiorly 12 mm superior to the symphysis pubis. The corset may be constructed of either nylon or cotton duck and usually is made with straps and buckles to allow the patient to adjust the abdominal compression. The corset extends to the lateral borders of the orthosis at the MATL. The corset may also be a stand-alone orthosis and is widely prescribed for low back pain. Corsets have been recorded as early as 1530 for Catherine of Medici.[2] Perry,[3] in her classic article on use of spinal orthoses found that the most often prescribed orthosis was the abdominal corset.

COMMONLY PRESCRIBED SPINAL ORTHOSES

Chair-Back LSO

The components of the chair-back orthosis are a pelvic band, a thoracic band, two paraspinal bars, and an abdominal corset or apron (Fig. 11–7). Biomechanically the orthosis is a combination of two three-point pressure systems. One system consists of

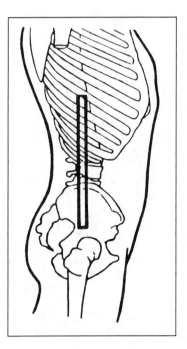

Figure 11–5. Lateral uprights, or bars. (Reproduced by permission from Berger, N, and Lusskin, R. Orthotic components and systems. In *American Academy of Orthopaedic Surgeons: Atlas of Orthotics.* St. Louis, Mo: Mosby; 1975.)

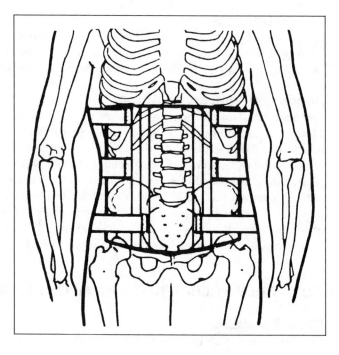

Figure 11–6. Abdominal support or apron. (Reproduced by permission from Berger, N, Lusskin, R. Orthotic components and systems. In: *American Academy of Orthopaedic Surgeons: Atlas of Orthotics*. St. Louis, Mo: Mosby; 1975.)

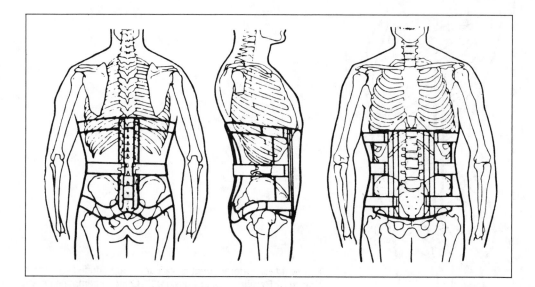

Figure 11–7. Chair-back LSO. (Reproduced by permission from Berger, N, Lusskin, R. Orthotic components and systems. In: *American Academy of Orthopaedic Surgeons: Atlas of Orthotics*. St. Louis, Mo: Mosby; 1975.)

two anteriorly directed forces from the thoracic and pelvic bands and a posteriorly directed force from the corset. The reverse is also true. There are two posteriorly directed forces from the corset and an anteriorly directed force from the paraspinal bars. Using these force systems, motions of lumbar flexion and extension are resisted, and the intraabdominal pressure is raised.

Raney LSO Flexion Jacket

Raney,[4] in 1969, reported on his experience with the Royalite flexion jacket. The orthosis that now bears his name (Fig. 11–8) was a by-product of the original Hauser flexion jacket, the first jacket used to flex the lumbar spine. The orthosis was developed by a patient who was an engineer with back pain and was fitted with a chair-back orthosis. Using a concave aluminum apron, the engineer added this new corset to the existing chair-back orthosis. Later orthoses were made of aluminum until Royalite was developed. Raney hypothesized that by flexing the lumbar spine, pressure was transferred to the anterior portion of the intervertebral disc, since the posterior portion of the disc was irritated in many cases. Results on over 1500 patients indicated that use of the Raney flexion jacket yielded relief of symptoms. The modern Raney flexion jacket is a custom-fitted spinal orthosis with a hard, anterior shell to maintain the lumbar spine flexed.

Knight LSO

The Knight LSO is very much like the chair-back except that in addition to the chair-back components, the Knight also has two lateral bars. Therefore in addition to the

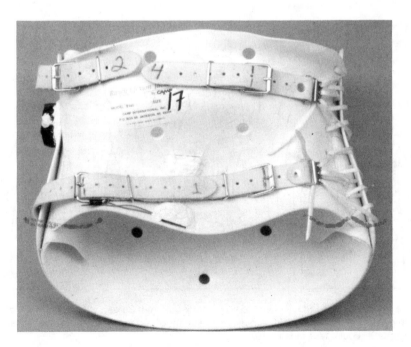

Figure 11–8. Raney flexion LSO.

three-point pressure systems of anteroposterior forces, there is limitation of lateral flexion via the lateral bars.

Williams LSO

The Williams LSO consists of a pelvic and thoracic band, a corset, and lateral/oblique bars (Fig. 11–9). These lateral/oblique bars allow the hinged orthosis to pivot on the thoracic band, thus allowing flexion of the lumbar spine and distal motion of the orthosis. Pulling on the anterior straps attached to both sides of the oblique bars causes the pelvis to be flexed and pulled anteriorly. The abdominal corset causes increased intraabdominal pressure to unload the lumbar spine.

In 1970 Perry[3] published the results of a study regarding the prescription of orthoses for spinal disorders. In this study chair-back and Knight LSOs were mentioned by 54% of the respondents and the Williams mentioned by 19%. No other orthosis was mentioned by more than 4.6% of the responses.

Jewett TLSO with Anterior Control

The Jewett hyperextension orthosis is composed of components that have not previously been discussed (Fig. 11–10). These components include a sternal pad and pubic pad anteriorly and a posteriorly located lumbar pad. The two anterior pads direct forces in the posterior direction, and the lumbar posterior pad directs one force anteriorly. This orthosis is used for patients who need to limit flexion or anterior motion following injury to the body of a vertebra, such as often occurs in a compression fracture. Since the Jewett has no lateral bars, there is little limitation to lateral bending.

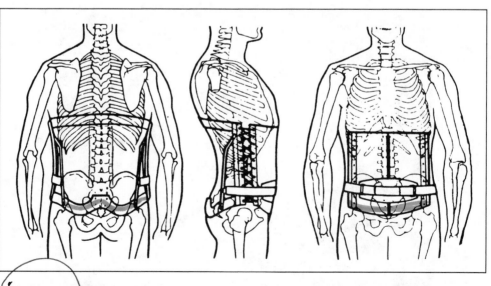

Figure 11–9. Williams LSO. (Reproduced by permission from Berger, N, Lusskin, R. Orthotic components and systems. In: *American Academy of Orthopaedic Surgeons: Atlas of Orthotics.* St. Louis, Mo: Mosby; 1975.)

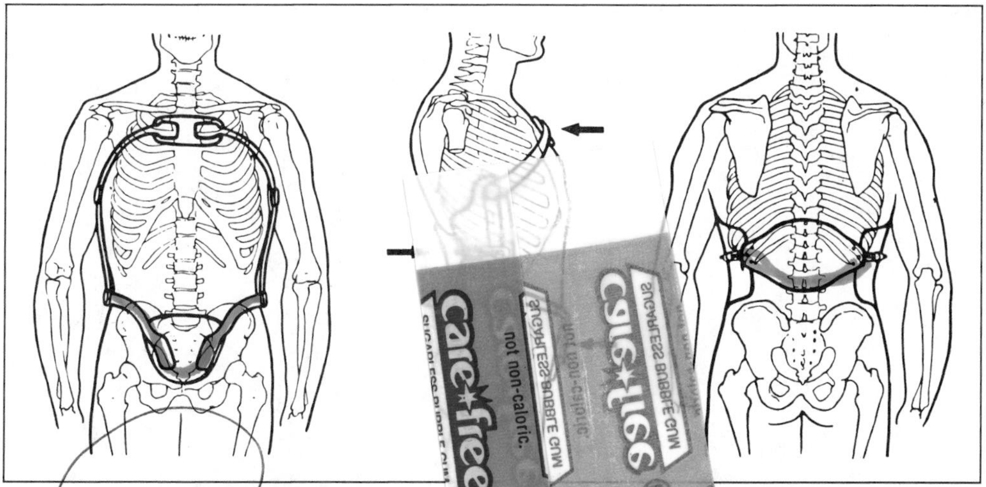

Figure 11–10. Jewett TLSO, anterior cor... ...ssion from Berger, N, and Lusskin, R. Orthotic components and ...n: ...Academy of Orthopaedic Surgeons: *Atlas of Orthotics*. St. Louis, M...

TLSO Body Jackets

The TLSO body jacket, which was former... ...d then iron and steel, is now made of plastic, either thermoplast... ...emoset plastics or acrylics (Fig. 11–11). These devices are either custom fabrica...ed from a model impression of each patient or custom fitted from prefabricated shells. ...set plastics have the advantage of being better contoured to the model but are more labor intensive and therefore more expensive.

Biomechanically TLSOs function similarly to other spinal orthoses but distribute forces over the largest possible area by using the principle of total contact. Depending on the amount of material removed from the model, the amount of intra-abdominal pressure may also be controlled. For many reasons TLSOs are the orthosis of choice for many patients. They may be washed, modified, and are quite cosmetic, being easily hidden under most loose-fitting clothes. TLSO body jackets may have either an anterior or posterior opening with velcro closures or may be bivalved, with straps on either side for easy entry and exit. Cotton T-shirts are often used to provide a comfortable interface between the plastazote lining and the skin. Cervical attachments may be added to TLSOs in cases of concomitant cervical spine injuries (Fig. 11–12).

Cervical Orthosis Components

Cervical orthoses do not have components in the same sense that thoracolumbar spinal orthoses do. Nachemson[5] makes a distinction between two groups of cervical orthoses: the cervical orthosis (CO) dealing with the region of C1-2; and the cervical thoracic orthosis (CTO) dealing with levels C-3 to T-1. Spinal kinematic studies suggest that flexion and extension occur mainly at the level of C5-6, while 80% of the rotation occurs

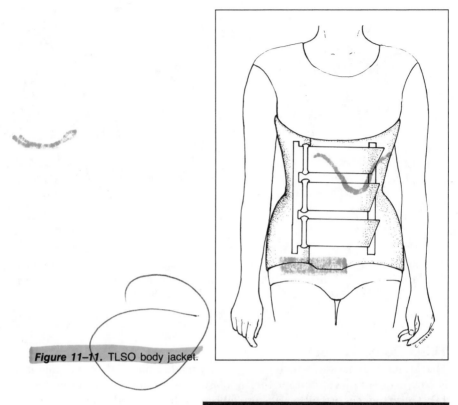

Figure 11–11. TLSO body jacket.

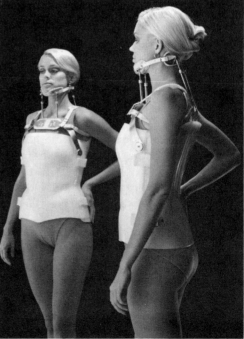

Figure 11–12. TLSO with cervical attachment. (From Becker Orthopaedic, Troy, Mich, with permission.)

at C1-2. This is borne out by a quick examination of the anatomy and the configuration of the cervical vertebrae.

A large percentage of cervical orthoses in use today are prefabricated. Nachemson[5] classifies cervical orthoses as soft, reinforced, or rigid. A soft cervical collar is usually made of polyurethane foam or foam rubber and is encased in a knitted material like stockinet. Rear closure is usually accomplished using Velcro.

The "Philadelphia" collar is an example of a reinforced cervical orthosis and is made of plastazote reinforced with plastic anteriorly and posteriorly (Fig. 11–13). These are available in 16 adult sizes and only recently available in pediatric sizes. Sizes are based on the distance from chin to chest and the circumference of the neck and are available with or without a cutout for an intubation tube. Another example of a reinforced cervical orthosis is the sternal-occipitomandibular immobilizer (SOMI; Fig. 11–14). The SOMI consists of three pieces: a sternal yoke, the anterior mandibular support, and the occipital support. These are easily fitted and are available in adult and pediatric sizes.

An example of a rigid cervical orthosis is the Halo (Fig. 11–15). Originally developed for polio patients, it has become widely used for the unstable cervical spine, usually at the C1-2 level, although it may be used for instability at inferior levels including the upper thoracic spine.

EFFECTS AND EFFECTIVENESS OF SPINAL ORTHOSES

In addition to the intended clinical functions of immobilization/motion control, support, and prevention/correction of skeletal deformity, several other consequences of the

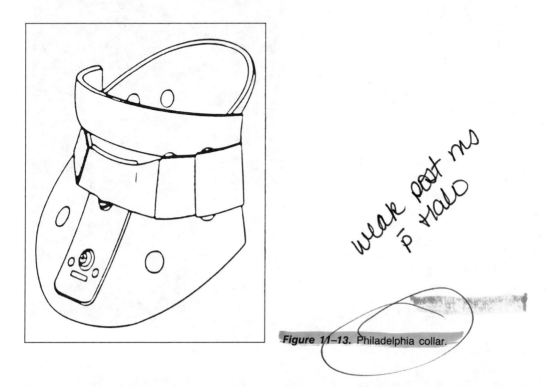

Figure 11–13. Philadelphia collar.

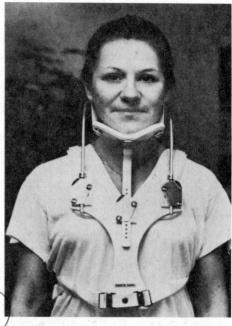

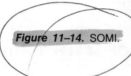

Figure 11–14. SOMI.

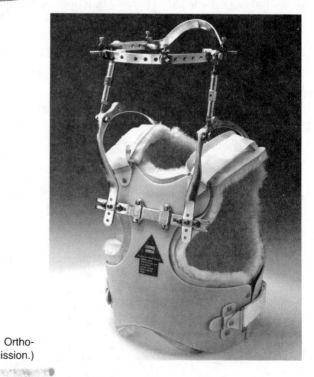

Figure 11–15. Halo. (From Fillauer Ortho-paedic, Chatanooga, Tenn, with permission.)

application of spinal orthoses have been described and/or studied. Not all effects of spinal orthotics are positive. Some negative effects are skin breakdown due to the intimate fit, psychologic dependency, weakened muscles, and aggravated symptoms, thought to be a by-product of inactivity or lack of motion. Reports of the effects and effectiveness of spinal orthoses are contained in the following sections.

Immobilization/Motion Control/Support

The normal anatomy of the human spine dictates to some extent what motions occur. For example, although there is motion of the thoracic spine, it is more limited than either the cervical or lumbar regions. Due to the thoracic spine construction, motion into flexion is greater than extension. Lateral bending of the spine increases as the spinal level moves inferiorly, but axial rotation decreases from superior to inferior. The lumbar spine allows flexion and extension but little pure rotation due to the construction and position of the facets.

White and Panjabi[6] refer to the "low stiff viscoelastic transmitter" when describing the medium between the orthosis and the skeletal structures of the spine. Because of the skin and soft-tissue interface, it is impossible for even the most rigid orthosis to completely immobilize the spine. To this end even the Halo has been shown by Johnson et al[7] to allow some cervical-spine motion. Since motion of bone at fracture sites is known to stimulate bone healing, some motion may be desirable in given orthotic applications. It remains the responsibility of the health care professional to understand the goal of each orthotic application to provide the best system consistent with the case.

Management of Thoracolumbar Fractures. Holdsworth[8] in 1963 was the first to use the term "burst fracture" to describe a spinal fracture caused by axial loading, causing the body of the vertebra to explode, thus threatening stability of the spine. The burst fracture may involve one or both of the bony end plates of the vertebral body and may or may not produce a loose bone fragment that can retropulse or move posteriorly to cause compression on the spinal cord and neurologic deficits.

In 1983 Denis[9] developed a three-part classification of spinal fractures. Instability of the first degree involves the risk of increasing kyphosis, as often seen in compression fractures. Such fractures may be treated with a TLSO spinal orthosis. Instability of the second degree involves a burst fracture with the prospect that further collapse of the fracture may lead to increased neurologic deficit. Denis believes that early ambulation or sitting even in a motion-limiting TLSO can cause further neurologic problems due to instability and axial loading. He reports on 20%, or 6 of 29, nonoperatively treated burst fractures without initial neurologic deficit who later developed deficits. Prior to Denis's[9] report, most fractures of thoracic and lumbar vertebrae were treated with either a TLSO or LSO with anterior control, using orthoses like the Jewett. In light of these findings, many surgeons have altered their postfracture treatment program to include a TLSO body jacket to control the fracture in all planes. The jacket is often lined with ¼ -in Plastazote to allow for minor changes in body size or configuration, since many of these patients wear their orthoses for 3 to 6 months and some longer. In cases where high thoracic and or concomitant cervical fractures occur, cervical extensions may be added to these orthoses without difficulty (Fig. 11–12). Most patients are able to don and doff the TLSO independently.

A recently published study from the University of Iowa found that neurologically intact burst fractures may be successfully treated nonoperatively using bed rest for six weeks followed by the use of a TLSO for up to six months (Weinsten J, personal communication 1988). According to this study there were no complications, and the occurrence of postinjury back pain or deformity was very small.

McEvoy and Bradford[10] reported a retrospective review of 399 fractures of the spine. Of these, 53 were followed for at least one year. All had burst fractures, 10 were thoracic, and 41 were lumbar. Thirty-eight had neurologic deficit, 22 of whom were treated nonsurgically and 31 operatively. The patients without deficit were treated with body jackets or casts and showed good results. At follow-up averaging three years, 68% were neurologically improved, although back pain was more common in the surgical group. These findings suggest that patients with burst fractures may be treated non-surgically with TLSO body jackets with good results.

Control of Thoracolumbar Spine Motion. Orthotic treatment intervention may be considered adjunctive and is often at least secondary; at worst it is used only after other treatments fail to provide the desired relief for soft-tissue or other disorders not surgically correctable. Fidler and Plasmans[11] in 1983 compared lumbosacral motion while using four spinal orthoses. These four orthoses were the canvas corset, the Raney LSO, the Baycast TLSO, and the Baycast TLSO with leg spica. Results indicated that the corset reduced the lumbar spine motion by one third; the Raney and Baycast TLSO reduced motion by two thirds; while the Baycast with spica was most effective. The Baycast with spica restricted angular movement below the third lumbar level as well as the lumbosacral junction. There was no restriction of the lumbosacral junction motion with only the LSOs or the Baycast jacket without spica. Therefore, if the orthotic goal is to reduce motion at the level of the lumbosacral junction, a TLSO with leg spica must be used.

To evaluate the role of primary orthotic treatment, J. Weinstein and K. Spratt (personal communication, 1988) reported on patients presenting with either spond-ylolisthesis or retrolisthesis who were randomly assigned to either a flexion or extension orthosis protocol. The method involved a very complete diagnostic evaluation to mea-sure spondy or retro displacement. This evaluation provided the baseline from which follow-up evaluations could be compared. A Raney flexion orthosis or TLSO with anterior control orthosis was randomly assigned and fitted by an experienced orthotist. Evaluation of treatment outcomes was assessed using a visual-analogue pain scale (VAS), a disability questionnaire (DQ), and the organic pain-behavior composite (OPBC). Results indicated that compliance of orthosis wearing was relatively good, with 60 of 65 (92%) returning for at least one of two follow-up visits. Even though only 55% of patients returned for both follow-up visits, 31 of 65 (48%) were found to be compliant, wearing the orthosis at least 100 h in one month or 400 h in four months. Females were found to be less compliant than males, although most of the females (eight of 10) were treated in flexion orthoses. None of the noncompliant subjects had been assigned an inappropriate orthosis, as judged by radiographic follow-up. A general tendency was for improvement over time, regardless of assignment protocol or amount of vertebral-body translation. Patients in extension orthoses demonstrated greater improvement as compared to all other patients for each of the three outcome criteria.

Cervical Spine Immobilization/Control. Soft collars provide kinesthetic reminders to immobilize the cervical spine. Hartman et al[12] reported that soft collars restrict only 5% to 10% of flexion and extension and provide no restriction to axial rotation. Johnson et al[13] studied 44 normal subjects wearing three of six possible cervical orthoses. These six were the soft collar, the Philadelphia collar, the four-poster orthosis, the SOMI, the Yale, and the Halo. Like Hartman et al,[12] Johnson et al[7] found the soft collar to be a useful reminder but little else. The Philadelphia collar was better than the soft collar but was not effective in controlling rotation. The four-poster orthosis, considered a CTO, was found to be equal to other CTOs in controlling flexion, especially of the middle cervical vertebrae. Similar to other CTOs, it was not effective in controlling rotation, lateral bending, and flexion and extension of the upper cervical spine. The other CTOs provided better fixation of the orthosis on the thorax and, thus, better cervical control. The Yale orthosis was the product of this study, since it was the best overall motion-restriction device tested, even though it lacked support at the C1-2 joint. Interestingly the SOMI was very successful at controlling motion at the C1-2 and C2-3 joints. Since the SOMI works well in controlling upper-level flexion, and since it is easily fitted in the supine position, it is often the orthosis of choice where upper cervical level flexion is a potential problem.

Johnson found the Halo, originally used at Rancho Los Amigos, to be the best overall orthosis in controlling rotation of the cervical spine, even though there was some motion measured even in the Halo. Because of the amount of distraction necessary to completely immobilize the spine and since acutely injured patients often cannot tolerate such distraction, there remains a bit of motion even with the Halo in place. The two clinical problems that can be associated with the Halo are pin loosening and infection. Lind et al (Lind BJ, Nordwall A, Sihlbom H, manuscript in preparation) studied the effects of the Halo orthosis on vital capacity. In neurologically intact patients, the Halo reduced the vital capacity by 10%, although the reduction was regained after removal of the Halo.

Deformity Prevention and Correction

The orthoses used for problems or diseases of the thoracic or thoracolumbar spine may either be TLSO or CTLSOs, depending on the nature of the pathology and its anatomic location. Perhaps the best known diseases treated with these orthoses are scoliosis and kyphosis. In these cases the orthoses act as a corrective device, applying forces in given directions to produce changes in the musculoskeleton.

The forces needed to correct a coronal plane deformity of the thoracic spine have been measured to be 3 to 5 kg. Andriacchi et al[14] demonstrated that the ribs provide stability, and this principle is used routinely with CTLSOs of the Milwaukee type (Fig. 11–16) by applying lateral superomedially directed forces with thoracic pads. This biomechanical model has been developed by Patwardhan et al[15] in a classic work that should be required reading for anyone involved in the management of these patients.

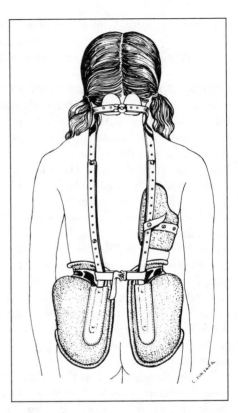

Figure 11–16. CTLSO, Milwaukee type.

Use of orthoses for idiopathic scoliosis and kyphosis is often based on the concept of active movement away from the pads, thus producing active correction. However, in neurologically based scolioses and kyphoses, patients may be unable to actively pull away from the pads, thus requiring a more passive treatment principle. CTLSOs and TLSOs are used in this patient group to allow supported sitting and to prevent further skeletal collapse. Radiographs of this patient group reveal "drooping ribs" that angle acutely and often nearly parallel to the bodies of the vertebrae. In these cases little support is provided by the lateral pads or lateral walls of the TLSO or body jacket. Generally the higher the apex of the cervical or thoracic curve the more difficult the control, the less effective the treatment, and the greater the chance of curve progression.

The literature in this area is ever evolving. There are critics who believe that many scoliotics are braced needlessly, since curve progression continues and surgical stabilization is eventually necessary. There are some who believe that most small curves (30 degrees or less) deserve careful observation and a trial using orthotic treatment. The natural history of scoliosis has yet to be completely elucidated. Retrospective studies show that about 30% of all idiopathic scoliotics will eventually arrest with no need for surgical stabilization. The clinical problem is how to prospectively determine who will arrest and who will progress and which treatment to provide. Weinstein and Ponseti[16] have written an excellent review on idiopathic scoliosis, indicating that double curves are at a greater risk for progression than single curves. The older the patient at presentation the less likely the progression. Curves detected before menarche tend to progress more than postmenarche, 66% to 33%. The lower the Risser sign at detection the greater the risk of progression. The larger the initial curve at detection the higher the risk.

Originally it was thought that once skeletal maturity was reached there was no further curve progression, although recent studies have demonstrated that this is not always the case. Weinstein and Ponseti[16] found that 68% of the curves in their study progressed after skeletal maturity unless they were less than 30 degrees. In thoracic curves the Cobb angle, apical vertebral rotation, and the Mehta angle were important prognostic factors. In lumbar curves the degree of apical vertebral rotation, the Cobb angle, the direction of the curve, and the relationship of the fifth lumbar vertebra to the intercrest line were of prognostic value. Curves that measured between 50 and 75 degrees at skeletal maturity, particularly thoracic curves, progressed the most, and average of one degree per year for 40 years. However, by further follow-up, these curves caused no more back pain than in the normal population and required no life-saving surgery or other procedures, as has been stated by some authors.

Weinstein and Ponseti[16] state that few long-term studies demonstrate brace effectiveness, since these studies do not document curve progression and since curve progression can be arrested orthotically in 85% to 90% of patients. The most common response to bracing is a moderate amount of correction while the orthosis is worn, with slow, steady progression of the curvature back to the original magnitude of the curve. This occurs, according to Weinstein and Ponseti,[17] in 80% of braced patients regardless of the curve pattern.

Miller et al[17] in 1984 reported on 255 patients aged 8 to 17 years with idiopathic scoliosis curves of 15 to 30 degrees. Divided into two groups, they were treated with CTLSO or no orthosis. Results showed a nonsignificant trend, suggesting that CTLSOs reduced the progression of the curve. However, since 75% of the curves were non-progressive, it is possible that no bracing would have been equally successful. The orthosis did prevent progression of 5% of the patients at a mean rate of 8% per year. Unfortunately these patients were not easily identified prospectively; thus, withholding treatment was not justified.

Gardner et al[18] discussed the search for prognostic indicators in the progression of scoliosis curves. The series of 70 unselected patients revealed that braced patients from 10 to 55 degrees did better than nonbraced. Best mean correction measured at 13 months following brace cessation was 41%. In the braced group, 33% progressed and 24% resolved by 5 degrees. Untreated patients progressed in 43% of cases, while 14% resolved by 5 degrees.

Winter et al[19] reported on 95 patients with thoracic curves of 30 to 39 degrees treated by CTLSOs from the same orthotic laboratory and treated with the same protocol. Follow-up averaged 2.5 years or until surgery. Of the 95, 15 (16%) eventually underwent surgery. For the 80 who did not, curve progression began at 33 degrees and at follow-up was 31 degrees. This reflects a pattern of similar studies but does not speak to the issue of difficult curves or curves that tend to progress in a high percentage of patients. A case report of a 57-degree T5-11 curve treated by brace is reported. Follow-up curve measured at 40 degrees. The authors suggest that no other explanations exists except that the CTLSO was effective.

Bassett and Bunnell[20] evaluated the influence of the axillary level Wilmington brace (Fig. 11–17) on spinal decompensation in adolescent idiopathic scoliosis. The concept of decompensation involves the relationship of a plumb line between the seventh cervical vertebra and the gluteal crease. The greater the distance between the two structures the greater the decompensation. Ideally, compensated curves will align over one another. Seventy-one patients with greater than 1 cm of decompensation were included in this study. Average follow-up was two years. There was no correlation between the Cobb angle pretreatment and the decompensation post-treatment. Results indicated that improvement averaged 1.4 cm for thoracic curves; 1.4 cm for thoracolumbar-lumbar; 1.5 cm for double-structural curves, with decompensation in 27 patients (38%) less than 1 cm. Six cases increased an average of 1.2 cm. The authors concluded that the Wilmington brace was successful in treating scoliosis.

The Rosenberger scoliosis orthosis (Fig. 11–18) is a low-profile, custom-molded orthosis used in the treatment of idiopathic scoliosis. It uses a snugly fitted end-support section and high counterforce trimlines on the concavity of the curve to aid the righting reflex. A corrective strap is located inside the jacket to reduce the curve by adding a transverse load in the posterolateral quadrant. Worn 23 h a day, it is used with apices below T6. Gavin et al[21] reported on 12 patients with curves averaging 25 to 35 degrees,

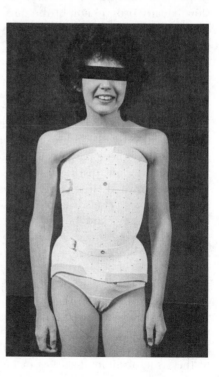

Figure 11–17. TLSO, Wilmington type. (Courtesy of Basset G, written communication, with permission.)

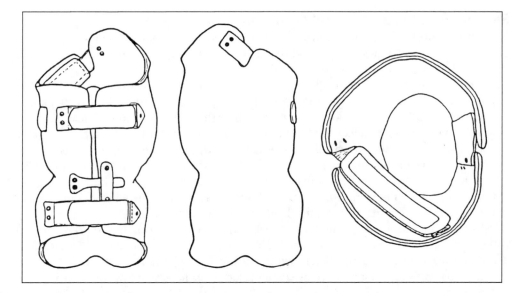

Figure 11–18. TLSO, Rosenberger. (**Left**) Anterior view of the orthosis, including trimline, opposition gradients, and high axillary wall. (**Middle**) Posterior trimline, with unique superior aspect. (**Right**) Transverse view, showing placement of corrective strap. (From: Gavin T, Bunch WH, Dvonch VM. The Rosenberger scoliosis orthosis. *J Assoc Child Prosthet/Orthot Clin.* 1986; **21**:37, with permission.)

mean 28.1 degrees. Initial reduction ranged from 23% to 100%, with a mean of 42.1%. Longer-term postbrace results were not presented.

Emans et al[22] reported on 295 patients treated with the Boston, low-profile TLSO system (Fig. 11–15) with at least one year postbracing follow-up. Prebrace curves ranged from 20 to 59 degrees using the Cobb method. Mean treatment time was 2.9 years. Mean best in-brace correction was 50%, with mean postbrace correction of 11%. Follow-up comparison with prebrace angles demonstrated 49% unchanged +/− 5 degrees, 39% correction of 5 to 15 degrees, 4% corrected 15 degrees or more, 4% lost 5 to 15 degrees, and 3% lost more than 15 degrees. Twelve percent eventually required surgery. An interesting point was stated relative to brace tolerance. The data indicated that partial brace compliance appeared as effective as full-time wearing. Emans et al[22] concluded that Boston orthoses without superstructure appeared as successful as with superstructure for curves with apices below T7.

Scheuermann's kyphosis, or epiphysitis, is a disease for which the literature indicates consistent successful orthotic treatment. Montgomery and Erwin[23] reviewed 203 cases of Scheuermann's kyphosis. Sixty-two wore Milwaukee type CTLSOs. Thirty-nine wore the orthosis for an average of 18 months. The mean curve was reduced from 62 degrees to 41 degrees. Further follow-up revealed a loss of correction of 15 degrees, indicating that 18 months of brace wearing was not enough.

Secondary Effects of Spinal Orthoses

Nachemson and Morris[24] studied in vivo effects of abdominal compression on intradiscal pressure. By using a very tight abdominal corset worn to the point of tolerance, intradiscal pressure was reduced by 30%.

Norton and Brown[25] inserted K wires into the spinous processes of lumbar vertebrae and posterosuperior iliac spines. Sitting was found to produce lumbar flexion of L5 and S1. Application of a long dorsal-lumbar orthosis focused forces near the T-L junction, too proximal to affect the lumbar spine. Flexion at the L5-S1 joint was greater in the orthosis, causing increased motion at the ends of the supported levels. These orthoses only reduced interspace flexion but did not eliminate it. While using an inflatable corset, the intradiscal pressure was lowered by 25%. This finding suggests that the clinical results using corsets and orthoses may be due partially to compression of the abdomen, thus decreasing the load on the vertebral column.

Waters and Morris[26] studied electrical activity of the trunk muscles with and without spinal orthoses. In standing, both a chair-back orthosis and corset caused decreased activity or had no effect, while during walking, neither orthosis had any effect. During fast walking there was increased muscle activity while wearing the orthoses.

THE FUTURE OF SPINAL ORTHOTICS

Undoubtedly future studies will continue to elucidate the important factors involved in the evaluation and treatment of disorders of the spine. With the use of improved imaging techniques, evaluation and follow-up will be more precise and specific. The role of nonsurgical interventions will be more thoroughly evaluated and understood, and as new materials and designs are developed, the place of spinal orthotics in the treatment regimen will become clearer.

REFERENCES

1. Lucas DB, Bresler B. Stability of the ligamentous spine. Technical Report No. 40, Biomechanics Laboratory, University of California, San Francisco and Berkeley, January 1961: 41.
2. Ewing E. *Fashion in Underwear.* London: Batsford; 1971.
3. Perry J. The use of external support in the treatment of low back pain. *J Bone Joint Surg.* 1970; **52A**:1440.
4. Raney FL. The royalite flexion jacket. *Spinal Orthotics.* Committee on Prosthetics Research and Development National Academy of Sciences. Monograph. 1969: 85.
5. Nachemson AL. Orthotic treatment for injuries and diseases of the spinal column. *Phys Med Rehabil.* 1987; 1(2):11–24.
6. White A, Panjabi M. *Clinical Biomechanics of the Spine.* Philadelphia, Pa: Lippincott; 1978.
7. Johnson RM, Hart DL, Simmons EF, Ramsby GR, Southwick WO. Cervical orthoses—A study comparing their effectiveness in restricting cervical motion in normal subjects. *J Bone Joint Surg.* 1977; **59A**:332.

8. Holdsworth FW. Fracture, dislocations, and fracture dislocations of the spine. *J Bone Joint Surg.* 1963; **45-B**:6.

9. Denis F. The three column spine and its significance in the classicification of acute thoracolumbar spinal injuries. *Spine.* 1983; 8:817.

10. McEvoy RD, Bradford DS. The management of burst fractures of the thoracic and lumbar spine. *Spine.* 1985; 10(7):631–637.

11. Fidler MW, Plasmans MT. The effect of four types of support on the segmental mobility of the lumbosacral spine. *J Bone Joint Surg.* 1983; 65A(7):943–947.

12. Hartman JT, Palumbo F, Hill BJ. Cineradiography of the braced normal cervical spine: A comparative study of five commonly used cervical orthoses. *Clin Orthop.* 1975; **109**:97–102.

13. Johnson RM, Owen JR, Hart DC, Callahan RA. Cervical orthoses: A guide to their selection and use. *Clin Orthop.* 1981; **154**:34,35.

14. Andriacchi T, Schultz A, Belytschco T, Galante J. A model for studies of mechanical interaction between the human spine and rib cage. *J Biomech.* 1974; **7**:497.

15. Patwardhan A, Vanderbs R, Knight GW, Gogan WJ, Levine PD. Biomechanics of the spine. In: Bund W, ed. *Atlas of Orthotics.* St. Louis, Mo: Mosby; 1985:139–150.

16. Weinstein SL, Ponseti IV. Curve progression in idiopathic scoliosis. *J Bone Joint Surg.* 1983; **65A**(4):447–455.

17. Miller JAA, Nachemson AL, Schultz AB. Effectiveness of braces in mild idiopathic scoliosis. *Spine.* 1984; 9(6):632.

18. Gardner ADH, et al. Some beneficial effects of bracing and a search for prognostic indicators in idiopathic scoliosis. *Spine.* 1986; **11**:779.

19. Winter RB, Lonstein JE, Drogt J, Noren CA. The effectiveness of bracing in the nonoperative treatment of idiopathic scoliosis. *Spine.* 1986; **11**:790,791.

20. Bassett GS, Bunnell WP. Influence of the Wilmington brace on spinal decompensation in adolescent idiopathic scoliosis. *Clin Orthop Rel Res.* 1987; **223**:164–169.

21. Gavin T, Bunch WH, Dvonch VM. The Rosenberger scoliosis orthosis. *Int Clin Info Bull.* 1986; **21**(3–4):35–38.

22. Emans JB, et al. The Boston bracing system for idiopathic scoliosis. *Spine.* 1986; 11(8):792–801.

23. Montgomery SP, Erwin WE. Scheuermann's kyphosis—long-term results of Milwaukee brace treatment. *Spine.* 1981; **6**(1):5–8.

24. Nachemson A, Morris JM. In vivo measurements of intradiscal pressure, a method for the determination of pressure in the lower lumbar disc. *J Bone Joint Surg.* 1964; **46A**:1077.

25. Norton PL, Brown T. The immobilizing efficiency of back braces. *J Bone Joint Surg.* 1957; **39A**:111–139.

26. Waters RL, Morris JM. Effects of spinal supports on the electrical activity of muscles of the trunk. *J Bone Joint Surg.* 1970; **52A**:51.

Index